Midwifery Revision

Midwifery Revision

OBJECTIVE AND OTHER TESTS FOR STUDENTS OF MIDWIFERY AND OBSTETRICS

Sarah E. G. Roch
SRN, SCM, MTD, FPA Certificate
Member of the English
National Board Midwifery Committee
Examiner to the English National Board for
Nursing, Midwifery and Health Visiting
Senior Midwifery Tutor,
Midwifery School, Princess Anne Hospital, Southampton

Foreword by Anne Bent
SRN, SCM, MTD
Lately Professional Officer (Midwifery)
UK Central Council
(Formerly Director of Education,
Royal College of Midwives)

THIRD EDITION

CHURCHILL LIVINGSTONE
EDINBURGH LONDON MELBOURNE AND NEW YORK 1986

CHURCHILL LIVINGSTONE
Medical Division of Longman Group UK Limited

Distributed in the United States of America by Churchill Livingstone Inc., 650 Avenue of the Americas, New York, N.Y. 10011, and by associated companies, branches and representatives throughout the world.

First edition 1980
Second edition 1983
Third edition 1986
Reprinted 1992

ISBN 0-443-03537-7

British Library Cataloguing in Publication Data
Roch, Sarah E. G.
Midwifery revision: objective and other tests for students of midwifery and obstetrics.— 3rd ed.
1. Obstetrics—Problems, exercises, etc.
I. Title
618.2'0076 RG532

Library of Congress Cataloging in Publication Data
Roch, Sarah E. G.
Midwifery revision.
Bibliography: p.
Includes index.
1. Obstetrics—Examinations, questions, etc.
2. Midwives—Examinations, questions, etc. I. Title.
[DNLM: 1. Midwifery—examination questions.
2. Obstetrics—examination questions. WQ 18 R672m]
RG532.R62 1986 618.2'0076 86-2274

The publisher's policy is to use **paper manufactured from sustainable forests**

Produced by Longman Singapore Publishers Pte Ltd
Printed in Singapore

Foreword

Examinations leading to qualifications which confer entry to a profession have inherent problems that are not always appreciated by those involved either as examiners or examinees. The final examinations of the midwives' statutory bodies are in this category. Examiners are required to ascertain that potential midwives have acquired the factual knowledge on which to base their practice.

Essay-type questions or conventional examinations are not necessarily the best way of testing factual knowledge although they may be used to test other attributes.

Miss Roch, in this book, is introducing students and teachers of midwifery to one possible solution by giving examples of objective tests to assess the level of factual knowledge of student midwives. The questions have been tested on a wide range of students and validated by computer, a process which is time-consuming and expensive but essential if this type of question is to be used for examination purposes.

The book is not, however, a haphazard introduction to objective testing; it is designed as a revision text for student midwives which is also very welcome.

Miss Roch qualified as a midwife teacher in 1969 and has taken a keen interest in educational developments and their place in midwifery education. It is therefore no surprise that she should have worked hard to produce this book which is the first of its kind for midwives to be published in the United Kingdom.

London, 1980 — Anne Bent

Preface to the Third Edition

Major statutory changes have taken place since the last edition of this book, with the inception of the UK Central Council and the National Boards for Nursing, Midwifery and Health Visiting replacing the previous nine statutory bodies under the Nurses, Midwives and Health Visitors Act 1979. Changes in the examination format have also taken place, and it now seems likely that more changes are on the way for the whole of the midwifery education system. This Third Edition has taken account of these alterations, and also added some new material. The book still provides a wide revision framework for students preparing for their midwifery qualifying examinations, and I hope that it will continue to help them.

Southampton, 1986 S.E.G.R.

Preface to the First Edition

This book has been compiled in the hope that it will help student midwives prepare for, and achieve success in their final Central Midwives Board examinations. Although at the present time objective tests do not form part of this examination system, a variety of these items are used here to introduce a wide range of subject matter, on which students can test their knowledge and reasoning ability. All these questions have been tested by a large group of student midwives from eight midwifery training schools, and then validated for item facility and discrimination at the Computer Centre, Moray House College of Education, Edinburgh.

The book is designed to be used as part of a planned revision programme, and besides the objective tests, practical suggestions are made on how to organise personal revision, plus advice on how to tackle the actual examinations.

Testing the objective items was a large task, and I am extremely grateful for the enthusiastic help I received from the tutorial staff and students of the Midwifery Schools at:

Barnsley District General Hospital
Greenwich and Bexley Area Health Authority
Jessop Hospital for Women, Sheffield
St Mary's Hospital, Newport, Isle of Wight
St Mary's Hospital, Portsmouth
Queen Charlotte's Hospital for Women
Odstock Hospital, Salisbury
Southampton General Hospital

I would also like to thank Mr P. J. Barker from Moray House Computer Centre, for his guidance, and the Central Midwives Board for their permission to publish questions from past examination papers.

My task has been made immeasurably easier by the efficient services of Miss Margaret King, who typed both the questions for testing, and the final manuscript with great precision.

Southampton, 1980 S.E.G.R.

For B. D. M.

Contents

Introduction— Planning revision and passing examinations

Midwifery is a very practical profession, and it is still an art, but with an increasingly scientific component. Unfortunately, in common with some other professions it is necessary to face the problem that examinations, based mainly on the theoretical aspects of the course, have to be passed before clinical skills can be practised. Therefore, success in the statutory written and oral examinations at the end of the course is as essential as becoming a capable and well-informed midwife.

Some people find theoretical study and examinations much easier than others, but for *everyone*, good preparation makes success far more certain. A common factor among the majority of those who have the misfortune to fail an examination is that both study and revision have been 'too little, too late'.

Revision

Let us look at the problems of revising for these particular examinations. There is no doubt that the present system demands the accurate recall of a considerable amount of theoretical knowledge, as well as its application to practical situations, so make a sensible and *realistic* revision plan at least 8–10 weeks before the examinations begin. Specialist and background knowledge will be sound if studying has been regular throughout the course, and books and journals have been read in addition to chosen basic textbooks. However, for a revision programme, it is probably wisest to use one's own lecture notes, and a familiar textbook.

During the last months of training, the emphasis is on abnormal midwifery and paediatrics, but remember that this training is preparation to become a practitioner of the *normal.* For this reason there have been many questions relating to normal midwifery and the role of the practising midwife in the final examination papers.

Towards the end of the course, many students go through a phase when they feel that they know *nothing.* Luckily this is rarely true! It is not possible to spend over a year in a busy maternity department and at least 3 months in the community, without acquiring a good deal of useful knowledge.

In these final weeks it is necessary to concentrate on organising and reviewing relevant knowledge already acquired, as only then can deficiencies be identified and remedied.

It is probable that some of the detail of subjects which were covered early in the course has been forgotten, for example, anatomy and physiology, normal pregnancy, labour and the puerperium and these should all be revised early on. Items such as statistics and social security benefits may alter frequently, and are difficult to remember for very long, so aim to look these up close to the examination, when the most up-to-date figures can be obtained.

Decide what subject matter will be revised each week. The 'mini-plans' which follow are a suggested frame-work only, and each individual student can rearrange, or add more detail to her own plan.

Plan 1

Week 1	Anatomy and Physiology	Uterus; tubes; ovary; urinary tract; bony pelvis; pelvic floor; male reproductive tract.
Week 2	Anatomy and Physiology	Menstrual/ovarian cycles; early development of fetus and placenta; mature placenta; fetal circulation; fetal skull.
Week 3	Pregnancy	Antenatal care; physiology of pregnancy; antenatal complications; medical disorders in pregnancy; fetal assessment.
Week 4	Labour	Physiology and management of normal labour; complicated labour.
Week 5	Puerperium	Physiology and management of normal puerperium; postnatal complications; multiple pregnancy.
Week 6	Neonatal Paediatrics	Physiology and management of the healthy neonate; infant feeding; the ill neonate; birth injury and congenital abnormalities.
Week 7	Miscellaneous	Family planning; drugs; antenatal education; social aspects of pregnancy.
Week 8	Community Health	National Health Service; Social Services; health legislation; statistics; maternity benefits; child health services; immunisation; 'children in care', etc.

Plan 2

Week 1	Anatomy of uterus, tubes and ovary; antenatal care and complications of pregnancy; maternity benefits; National Health Services.
Week 2	Early development of fetus and placenta; the mature placenta; placental function tests; fetal assessment; social aspects of pregnancy; non-accidental injury in children.
Week 3	Anatomy of breast and physiology of lactation; physiology and management of the normal baby; infant feeding; immunisation programmes.
Week 4	Menstrual and ovarian cycles; physiology and management of normal labour; fetal circulation; birth asphyxia; resuscitation; social aspects of pregnancy.

Week 5	Anatomy of pelvic floor and male reproductive tract; the puerperium — normal and complicated; neonatal jaundice; family planning.
Week 6	The fetal skull; birth injuries; congenital abnormalities; Health and Social Services; provision for children in the community.
Week 7	The bony pelvis and pelvic assessment; complicated labour; obstetric emergencies; care of the ill and immature neonate.
Week 8	Anatomy of the urinary tract; urinary tract problems in pregnancy, labour and puerperium; health legislation and statistics; sexually transmitted diseases.

Having made a plan, decide whether to do a little work each day, or set aside so many evenings or days each week. *Write out the plan*, and stick it up on the wall where it can be easily seen. Tick each section off as it is completed, and this part at least will be a source of encouragement!

Each student should consider whether she studies better on her own, with a friend, or in a small group, and decide if it is easier to work in a library, in her own room, or in a communal room. It needs real self-discipline to shut oneself away and study when friends seem to be enjoying themselves, but if one is strong-willed it will soon be possible to taste the fruits of victory.

The examinations

The examination format has been revised for the extended midwifery education and training courses, and now consists of two 3-hour written papers and a 20-minute oral examination conducted by an approved examiner who is an experienced midwife teacher.

Two other midwife teacher examiners mark the written papers, and so each candidate is examined by three separate examiners.

The two written papers *both* cover the full range of relevant knowledge and clinical practice relating to both hospital and community, which the student will have experienced within the curriculum.

Each paper will consist of six questions. The first five will be 'essay-type' questions and the candidate will choose three to answer, and should allocate approximately 45 minutes to each answer. Question 6 will consist of eight topics from which the candidate will select four, and should allocate approximately 7–10 minutes to each short answer.

All the questions are 'weighted' so that the candidate can see not only the total marks allotted for each question, but also, where it is appropriate, the allocation of marks to different parts of a question, for example:

	Marks
Describe the anatomy of the breast.	20
What measures can a midwife take to:	
a. encourage women during the antenatal period to breast feed?	40
b. provide support for women who are breast feeding?	40
	100

Define pre-term labour.	10
Outline the role of the midwife providing care during pre-term labour.	40
List the more common complications which may occur in a baby born at 36 weeks gestation.	20
Describe *briefly* how these complications could be managed.	30
	100

This can be very helpful to the examinee when deciding on *timing* and *emphasis* in answering the question.

The onus is on the *student* to convince her examiners that she has achieved a satisfactory standard of knowledge and clinical expertise which will enable her to practise safely as a midwife. The examiners have every right to expect proof that the candidate can give a good standard of care in all practical procedures, especially those which directly affect the well-being of the mother and her baby. Therefore, every student should be particularly well-informed on all aspects of patient care, and what action a midwife would take in emergency situations such as postpartum haemorrhage, cord prolapse, severe birth asphyxia etc. Wherever possible, *personal practical experience* should be used, rather than trying to remember vast tracts of textbook material. Every student should train herself to recall procedures actually seen and done. It is generally easier to remember what treatment was used for 'Jenny Jones in Bed 3, who had an antepartum haemorrhage', than to recollect what was on 'page 317' in one's textbook.

The written examination

There are certain points which may help the student to communicate her considerable knowledge and clinical competence to the examiners. Firstly, although this is not an examination in the skills of the English language, there is no doubt that legible handwriting, understandable grammar, and *some* punctuation will improve the presentation of examination material. A reasonable standard of spelling is also important, as technical words and drug names must be accurate on reports and treatment charts.

Secondly, a tidy, well-spaced answer with suitable headings and sub-headings (where appropriate) makes a paper much easier to read and evaluate, and is appreciated by examiners.

These are all items which improve with practice and planning, so it is of value to use the selection of questions from past examination papers, which are at the end of each chapter.

For the final examination, it may be helpful to consider the following points:

1. Read the whole paper through carefully.

2. When planning each individual answer, underline the important *key words* in the question. For example:
   'Following a period of *unsatisfactory intra-uterine growth*, a baby is born at *36 weeks'* gestation. Describe the *care* that may be necessary during the *first week of life.*'

   In the short questions too, this can be useful. When asked to write briefly on 'The *diagnosis* of *breech* presentation in *labour*', it was amazing how many students actually wrote about breech *delivery* or *prenatal* diagnosis! It is extremely easy to make mistakes under stress, and underlining the key words may help to avoid this particular pitfall, and ensure that each question in properly understood.

3. *Essay questions*
   Essay questions make up the longest section of each written paper, and all will relate to the midwife's role and professional responsibilities. 45 minutes are allocated for each of the 3 questions to be answered, and this time must include a few minutes for choosing wisely, thinking and planning.

   These answers should have a clearly defined introduction to the subject followed by the main body or substance of the answer, and finally a conclusion. Sub-headings may or may not be helpful, and should only be used if they organise and clarify your information. The format of these questions varies, and it is important that they are correctly interpreted. For example, if asked to 'discuss' a subject, the student should state all the points 'for' and 'against', and if appropriate, draw positive conclusions. The term 'describe' indicates that a full and detailed account of the subject should be given, and this can include making a simple drawing or diagram.

   If the question requires one to make a 'list', items should be written down in a sensible, logical order, while 'enumerate' indicates that the answer material is to be presented in a numbered format, i.e. 1, 2, 3 etc. The term 'state' asks one to set out clearly, specific information about a topic, and 'define' is to explain the exact meaning or nature of the subject as succinctly as possible.

4. *Short questions*
   These questions are often extremely challenging, as they require the student to select facts that are both important and relevant from a body of information, and it is frequently difficult to decide what is *most* significant when faced with a large number

of facts. In many cases it is helpful for the student to ask herself 'what is of greatest importance about the subject to a practising midwife?', and then to write a brief explanatory paragraph about each chosen item. The short time-allowance of only 7–10 minutes makes it imperative to be both brief and concise.

5. Plan each answer *very briefly* on rough paper, and then use the headings to write it out in detail. Decide whether the answer needs a detailed definition, or if there are any appropriate headings or sub-headings that could be used. For example:

Diagnosis	Pregnancy
Signs and symptoms	Labour
Causes	Puerperium
Incidence	Maternal
Causative organism	Fetal
Medical management	Mother
Nursing care	Baby
Drug therapy	First stage
Complications	Second stage
Dangers	Third stage
Contra-indications	
Prevention	
Prognosis	

6. *Timing.*
   This is *vital* for success. In practice, and in the real examination, it is important to take only the correct time allowance [i.e. essay-type questions (45 minutes) and short questions (approximately 7–10 minutes)]. If this is exceeded, questions may be left out, or answered briefly and badly. Even if one or two questions have been answered really well, it will not compensate for omissions, or several answers of a poor standard. If you need extra time for answer planning, take it from the time allowed for the *long* answers *not* the short ones. Aim for *consistency*. One does not have to be brilliant to pass; a steady, competent display will do very well.

   Students who persistently overrun their time allowance should consult their tutors who will give them individual help to select important points and condense information, which may save valuable minutes.

   Discard all irrelevant material ruthlessly. No matter how good it may be, it will not gain any credit in the examination, and may even lead to the omission of vital facts for lack of time.

7. Students who write slowly may find tabulation helpful, as credit is given for *facts*, and not necessarily for flawless prose!.

8. Make sure that all information is in a sensible order, with commonly occurring matter first, and rarely-seen items at the end of the list.

9. Remember that one gets tired towards the end of a long paper, and most people slow down during the last half hour of an examination. If one falls behind early on, the last questions may have to be hurried, and this will leave no time at the end to check for obvious errors.

10. In general, abbreviations are best avoided, especially obscure ones, but those in common use are acceptable, (e.g. BP for blood pressure). When used, the full term should be written out initially with the abbreviation in brackets beside it, and after this the abbreviation alone may be written each time, (e.g. artificial rupture of membranes (A. R. M.)).

11. When attempting a diagram, (and for demonstrating anatomy they are very worthwhile), make it *big*, coloured and well-labelled. The information need not be repeated in words, as diagrams should be simple, and save both words and time.

    Lastly, *think positively and practically*, and the battle is half won.

The oral examination

Many students find this part of the examination more stressful than the written papers, because they have to travel to London, or a regional centre, and meet unknown people in a strange environment. Everyone is tense and anxious, but being well-prepared will boost one's confidence.

Before setting out for the oral examination, all students should check they have their examination card, and arrive in good time, looking neat and professional, but comfortable too.

It is important to remember that examiners are more likely to ask about practical midwifery knowledge and care, rather than obscure abnormalities.

On entering the examination room most people feel terribly nervous, but *do smile* and greet your examiners pleasantly. Examiners *are* human, and really do want all students to reach the standard required for success! Unfortunately, they have not seen the candidates at work in the wards and departments, and so have to rely on the written papers, and this 20 minute face-to-face encounter, for evidence that the student is a safe practical midwife.

It may be hard when you are apprehensive but do try to look the examiner straight in the eye, speak clearly, and don't fiddle, or display other irritating mannerisms. Most of us do something odd under stress. If handed a doll and pelvis, *do use it*. Don't just sit there clutching it!

This oral examination gives the student a great chance to communicate her hard-won knowledge and attitudes, and may well provide the opportunity to redeem errors or omissions from the written papers.

Finally, every candidate should concentrate on what she *knows*; utilise her own clinical experience, and if asked for an opinion, be confident enough to express a personal view.

Suggestions on how to use this book

This book is designed to assist you to revise subject matter covered during your midwifery training. A wide range of material is brought to your attention by using a number of objective and other tests. The answers, and in many cases some additional explanation, are easily available on the page following the questions. These tests will help you to decide what you know, and how much further information you need. Questions are generally in a random order, which is intentional, and it should make your mind more flexible, and capable of moving quickly from one subject to another.

You may think that some of the questions have a 'trick' answer, but this is not the intention, and you will usually find upon reflection, that reading the question more carefully would have prevented you from giving an incorrect response. This will train you to read all questions with great care, and perhaps save you from making a similar mistake in the examinations, which could penalise you severely.

MULTIPLE CHOICE QUESTIONS

Single response
In these questions there is an initial statement, (called the stem), followed by *four* alternative responses, only *one* of which is correct.

Multiple response
Here the stem is followed by five alternative responses, any number of which between 1–5 may be correct.

True or false?
For these items you must indicate whether you consider the statement to be correct or incorrect.

Matching items
In these tests there are two groups of items, and each of the *four* Group 1 items have to be matched with *one* of the *five* Group 2 items, with which it will have a strong association.

Assertion/reason
These items are a particular test of your reasoning ability, as you

not only have to decide whether or not each statement is true or false, but whether the reason is the *correct* reason for the initial statement.

Completion items
Here you simply fill in the missing word or words in each statement.

You will find an example of how to answer each type of question at the beginning of each section in Chapter 1.

Don't attempt to answer *all* the questions in quick succession, but tackle a few at a time, and note down any subjects you need to revise further. Use the past examination questions at the end of each chapter to practise preparing answers, and as a reminder for additional revision.

Finally, at the end of the book, you will find a short list of books which you may find useful for further reference and revision.

1. Anatomy and physiology

SECTION 1
SINGLE RESPONSE MULTIPLE CHOICE QUESTIONS

Questions 1.1–1.37
Select a *single* correct response to each of the following questions:

Example: **The non-pregnant uterus weighs:**
A 30 g
B 60 g
C 100 g
D 120 g

Answer: **B** (60 g)

1.1 The lining of the non-pregnant uterus is called the:
A myometrium
B parametrium
C endometrium
D decidua

1.2 The lining of the pregnant uterus is the:
A myometrium
B decidua
C endometrium
D parametrium

1.3 The acid reaction of the vagina is caused by:
A hydrochloric acid
B sodium carbonate
C lactic acid
D carbonic acid

1.4 Human milk is produced in the breasts by:
A acini cells
B myo-epithelial cells
C lactiferous tubules
D transitional epithelium

(*answers overleaf*)

1.1 **C**

1.2 **B**

1.3 **C**

1.4 **A**

1.5 The blood normally contains:
A 5000–10 000 leucocytes per cu mm
B 50 000–100 000 leucocytes per cu mm
C 500–1000 leucocytes per cu mm
D 5 million eosinophils per cu mm

1.6 Maintenance of blood pressure is dependent upon:
A activity
B partial pressure of oxygen
C peripheral resistance
D the bundle of His

1.7 The lateral sinuses from the tentorium cerebelli drain into the:
A great vein of Galen
B circle of Willis
C cisterna magna
D internal jugular veins

1.8 Spermatozoa are produced in the:
A prostate gland
B testes
C seminal vesicle
D vas deferens

1.9 Which of the following muscles principally supports the vagina?
A bulbocavernosus
B ischiocavernosus
C transverse perinei
D gluteus medius

1.10 Ovulation occurs:
A after the formation of the corpus luteum
B 14 days prior to menstruation
C in response to follicle stimulating hormone
D 14 days after menstruation

1.11 Fertilisation of the ovum usually takes place in:
A the ampulla of the uterine tube
B the infundibulum
C the uterine cavity
D the interstitial portion of the uterine tube

1.12 The secretory phase of the menstrual cycle refers to:
A the phase prior to ovulation
B the phase prior to menstruation
C the ovulatory phase
D the menstrual phase

(*answers overleaf*)

1.5 **A**

1.6 **C**
This is the variable pressure exerted throughout the peripheral circulation, by the arterioles, whose vessel walls contain smooth muscle fibres.

1.7 **D**

1.8 **B**

1.9 **A**

1.10 **B**
Ovulation occurs in response to the production of luteinizing hormone by the anterior pituitary gland.
The second half of the menstrual cycle is comparatively stable. It is the *first half* that varies when the woman has a long or a short cycle.

1.11 **A**

1.12 **B**

1.13 The functional unit of the ovary after puberty is the:
- **A** primordial follicle
- **B** corpus luteum
- **C** Graafian follicle
- **D** luteal cell

1.14 The ovarian cycle is under the influence of:
- **A** the endometrium
- **B** the cerebral cortex
- **C** the anterior pituitary gland
- **D** the posterior pituitary gland

1.15 Lutein cells are found in:
- **A** Bowman's capsule
- **B** spermatocytes
- **C** tunica adventitia
- **D** corpus luteum

1.16 Which of these hormones directly control ovarian function:
- **A** oestrogen and progesterone
- **B** follicle stimulating hormone and progesterone
- **C** oestrogen and luteinising hormone
- **D** follicle stimulating hormone and luteinising hormone

1.17 The basic functional unit of the mature placenta is:
- **A** syncitium
- **B** chorionic villus
- **C** mesoderm
- **D** trophoblast

1.18 The placenta is made up of 18–20 lobes, divided by small fissures. These lobes are called:
- **A** chorionic villi
- **B** parietes
- **C** alveoli
- **D** cotyledons

1.19 The small fissures between the lobes of the placenta are called:
- **A** raphes
- **B** sulci
- **C** gyri
- **D** lacunae

(*answers overleaf*)

1.13 **C**

1.14 **C**

1.15 **D**

1.16 **D**
Follicle stimulating hormone ripens the Graafian follicle, and luteinising hormone is involved to the process leading to ovulation.

1.17 **B**
Chorionic villi may be either *anchoring* villi, or (more numerous) *nutritive* villi. The syncytium (or syncytiotrophoblast) and the cytotrophoblast (Langhan's layer) are the outer layers of the villus wall, which are derived from the original trophoblast.

1.18 **D**

1.19 **B**

1.20 The bones which form the vault of the fetal skull are laid down in:

A membrane
B cartilage
C fibrous tissue
D reticular tissue

1.21 The vertex is the region bounded by:

A mentum, glabella and malar bones
B glabella, anterior fontanelle and temporal bones
C parietal eminences, anterior fontanelle and occipital protuberance
D anterior and posterior fontanelles, and parietal eminences

1.22 The double fold of dura mater lying between the two cerebral hemispheres is called the:

A hypothalamus
B falx cerebri
C basal ganglia
D tentorium cerebelli

1.23 The fold of dura mater between the cerebrum and the cerebellum, is called the:

A hypothalamus
B tentorium cerebelli
C falx cerebri
D basal ganglia

1.24 The venous blood from much of the brain is collected into a large vessel called the____________________, which then joins the straight sinus at the junction of the falx cerebri and the tentorium cerebelli:

A external jugular vein
B internal jugular vein
C circle of Willis
D great vein of Galen

1.25 The acidity of the vagina is maintained by the action of saprophytic organisms on glycogen contained in the cells of the vaginal epithelium. These organisms are named:

A Köch's bacilli
B Ducrey's bacilli
C Döderlein's bacilli
D Streptokinase

(*answers overleaf*)

1.20 **A**
The majority of the skeletal structure in man is laid down in cartilage, but the vault bones are laid down in membrane, so that the sutures and fontanelles can be formed, which allow moulding to take place during labour.

1.21 **D**

1.22 **B**

1.23 **B**

1.24 **D**

1.25 **C**

1.26 The vagina has a lining of:
A stratified epithelium
B columnar epithelium
C squamous epithelium
D cubical epithelium

1.27 The lower uterine segment is formed from:
A the cervix
B the cornua
C the corpus
D the isthmus

1.28 A line drawn between the inferior border of the symphysis pubis and the sacral promontory is known as the:
A diagonal conjugate
B true conjugate
C anatomical conjugate
D curve of Carus

1.29 The pelvic brim inclines at an angle of approximately:
A 55°
B 60°
C 65°
D 70°

1.30 In a gynaecoid pelvis, the smallest diameter of the pelvic outlet is:
A bituberous
B bispinous
C antero-posterior
D oblique

1.31 The naturally occurring pelvic type with a characteristic flat brim is called:
A anthropoid
B platypelloid
C rachitic
D android

1.32 Prominent ischial spines and a narrow sub-pubic arch are associated with a:
A gynaecoid pelvis
B anthropoid pelvis
C android pelvis
D platypelloid pelvis

(*answers overleaf*)

1.26 **C**

1.27 **D**

The isthmus is the narrow band of corpus uteri adjoining the internal os which expands during pregnancy to form the lower uterine segment.

1.28 **A**

The diagonal conjugate can be assessed on pelvic examination. The true conjugate is measured from the centre of the sacral promontory to the upper border of the symphysis pubis. It may also be called the anatomical conjugate. The obstetrical conjugate is a practical measurement of value to the clinician. It is measured between the sacral promontory and the *inner* border of the symphysis pubis, and indicates the actual space available for the fetus.

1.29 **A**

1.30 **B**

1.31 **B**

1.32 **C**

1.33 Cerebro-spinal fluid is produced by:
- **A** pia mater
- **B** plexus of Lee-Frankenhauser
- **C** dura mater
- **D** choroid plexus

1.34 Testosterone is secreted by:
- **A** the adrenal medulla
- **B** prostate gland
- **C** interstitial cells of the testes
- **D** seminal tubules

1.35 The function of the prostate gland is to:
- **A** produce spermatozoa
- **B** secrete testosterone
- **C** produce norethisterone
- **D** secrete lubricant for spermatozoa

1.36 The large bowel contains bacteria as its normal flora, which synthesise:
- **A** vitamin B
- **B** vitamin A
- **C** vitamin E
- **D** vitamin K

1.37 The choroid plexus lies in the:
- **A** cisterna magna
- **B** lateral ventricles
- **C** extra-dural space
- **D** fourth ventricle

(*answers overleaf*)

1.33 **D**

1.34 **C**

1.35 **D**

The prostate gland secretes a lubricant fluid rich in acid phosphatase into the urethra. It dilutes the seminal fluid and aids the mobility of the spermatozoa.

1.36 **D**

Vitamin K is necessary for the production of prothrombin in the liver. Some vitamin K is acquired in the diet (e.g. green vegetables, carrots etc.) and the remainder is synthesised by the normal flora of the large bowel.

1.37 **B**

A choroid plexus is situated in the roof of each of the two lateral ventricles of the cerebral hemispheres, and these capillary networks produce cerebrospinal fluid. In immature infants lethal intraventricular haemorrhage may occur involving these structures.

SECTION II
MULTIPLE RESPONSE QUESTIONS Questions 1.38–1.73

Select any number of correct responses between 1–5

Example: **The landmarks on the pelvic brim include:**
- **A** sacral promontory
- **B** ilio-pectineal line
- **C** obturator foramen
- **D** sacrospinous ligament
- **E** symphysis pubis

Answer: **A B E**

1.38 The uterus:
- **A** weighs approximately 600 g in the non-pregnant state
- **B** forms its lower segment from the isthmus in late pregnancy
- **C** is normally retroverted in early pregnancy
- **D** receives its main blood supply from the ovarian and uterine arteries
- **E** contracts painlessly during pregnancy

1.39 The cervix:
- **A** has a junction of squamous and columnar epithelium
- **B** contains a well-formed canal
- **C** has an internal and an external os
- **D** secretes acid mucus
- **E** secretes alkaline mucus

1.40 The structures supporting the uterus are:
- **A** cardinal ligaments
- **B** pelvic floor
- **C** utero-sacral ligaments
- **D** pubo-cervical ligaments
- **E** broad ligaments

1.41 The Fallopian (uterine) tubes:
- **A** are each attached to an ovary by an ovarian fimbria
- **B** may be the site of an ectopic pregnancy
- **C** are lined with ciliated epithelium
- **D** are enclosed by the round ligaments
- **E** convey ova to the uterine cavity

(*answers overleaf*)

1.38 **B D E**
The non-pregnant uterus weighs approximately 60 g and is normally anteflexed and anteverted.

1.39 **A B C E**

1.40 **A B C D**
The two cardinal ligaments (also known as the transverse cervical or Mackenrodt's ligaments) extend from the lateral aspect of the cervix, just below the internal os, to the side walls of the pelvis. The broad ligaments are not *true* ligaments, but merely a double fold of pelvic peritoneum which envelops the uterine tubes.

1.41 **A B C E**
The tubes are enclosed by the *broad* ligaments.

1.42 The ovary:
A is situated on the anterior aspect of the broad ligament
B is attached to the uterus by the ovarian ligament
C contains Graafian follicles embedded in its medulla
D has an excellent blood supply from the ovarian artery
E is supplied by autonomic nerve fibres from the plexus of Lee-Frankenhauser

1.43 The vagina:
A is lined by squamous epithelium
B is an alkaline medium
C is lined by columnar epithelium
D forms the four fornices at its upper end
E contains Bartholin's glands

1.44 The broad ligament contains:
A ovary
B ovarian artery and vein
C ureter
D round ligament
E Fallopian tube

1.45 The bladder:
A receives autonomic nerve supply from the plexus of Lee-Frankenhauser
B contains the detrusor muscle
C has a normal capacity of approximately 500–600 ml
D can overdistend to hold 1–2 litres of urine
E is lined by transitional epithelium

1.46 The trigone of the bladder:
A contains muscle fibres running between the two ureteric orifices, known as Mercier's bar
B is situated in the apex of the bladder
C has muscle fibres running from the ureteric orifices to the internal meatus, called the muscles of Bell
D contains Bell's muscles which open the internal urinary meatus during the act of micturition
E has its epithelial surface thrown into folds, called rugae, which allow for distension

1.47 The female breast:
A is an exocrine gland
B is also called the mammary apparatus
C contains milk-producing alveolar tissue
D contains a considerable amount of fat
E enlarges at puberty

(*answers overleaf*)

1.42 **B D E**
The ovaries are situated on the *posterior* aspect of the broad ligament, and the Graafian follicles are embedded in the ovarian *cortex*.

1.43 **A D**
The vagina is an *acid* medium, and only receives the duct openings from Bartholin's glands at its introitus.

1.44 **B C D E**
The ovary lies *outside* the broad ligament, on its posterior aspect.

1.45 **A B C D E**

1.46 **A C D**
The trigone is the triangular shaped *base* of the bladder, and its lining of transitional epithelium is *not* thrown into folds as is the rest of the bladder epithelium.

1.47 **A B C D E**

1.48 Which of the following factors is *not* an essential factor in blood coagulation:

A fibrinogen
B thromboplastin
C vitamin B_{12}
D calcium
E glycogen

1.49 Blood:

A has a pH 7.4 (approx.)
B contains 5–6 000 000 red blood cells/cu mm
C has a decreased white cell count in pregnancy
D should have a haemoglobin level of 11–12 g/dl in pregnancy
E has a decreased platelet count in pregnancy

1.50 The red blood cells in iron deficiency anaemia are described as:

A microcytic
B macrocytic
C megaloblastic
D hyperchromic
E hypochromic

1.51 The placenta produces:

A oestrogens
B progesterone
C chorionic gonadotrophin
D human placental lactogen
E steroids

1.52 The function of the placenta is to:

A provide active transfer of nutrients
B excrete urea and other waste products
C allow diffusion of oxygen and carbon dioxide
D prevent the passage of all pathogenic organisms
E store and mobilise glycogen

1.53 Which of the following statements about the umbilical cord is correct?

A contains two arteries
B it contains two veins
C oxygenated blood is carried in a vein
D maternal blood is carried in the umbilical arteries
E Wharton's jelly has a protective function

(*answers overleaf*)

1.48 **C E**

1.49 **A B D**
Both the platelet and the white cell counts usually increase during pregnancy.

1.50 **A E**
The red cells are pale (hypochromic) and small and immature (microcytic).

1.51 **A B C D E**

1.52 **A B C E**
Some organisms (e.g. spirochaete of syphilis), and most viruses are able to cross the placenta to the fetus.

1.53 **A C E**
The single umbilical vein carries oxygenated blood to the fetus from the placenta. The fetal circulation contains only fetal blood, and under normal circumstances fetal and maternal blood do not mix.

1.54 The function of Wharton's jelly is to:
- **A** provide nutrition for the fetus
- **B** protect the umbilical vessels from damage
- **C** produce gammaglobulin
- **D** excrete waste products from the fetus
- **E** keep the umbilical vessels patent

1.55 The formation of amniotic fluid is not fully understood, but it is thought to come from the following sources:
- **A** diffusion through the umbilical cord
- **B** secretion from the decidua
- **C** fetal urine
- **D** transudate from the amnion
- **E** fluid from the fetal lungs

1.56 Amniotic fluid:
- **A** in early pregnancy resembles maternal plasma
- **B** contains protein
- **C** contains fetal urine after about 20 weeks
- **D** acts as a shock absorber for the fetus
- **E** is bacteriocidal

1.57 In the normal fetal circulation:
- **A** the ductus venosus connects the umbilical vein with the inferior vena cava
- **B** the two hypogastric arteries are continuous with the two umbilical arteries
- **C** the two ventricles communicate through a septal defect
- **D** the foramen ovale connects the two atria
- **E** the ductus arteriosus connects the pulmonary vein with the aorta

1.58 Human spermatozoa:
- **A** enter the vas deferens when they leave the testes
- **B** when mature have only 23 chromosomes
- **C** contain hyaluronidase
- **D** are motile at ejaculation
- **E** are about 50 microns in length

1.59 The innominate bone:
- **A** has three constituent bones which fuse in the acetabulum
- **B** consists of pubis, ischium, and sacrum
- **C** has a synovial joint between the two pubic bones
- **D** meets the sacrum at the sacro-iliac joint
- **E** contains the obturator foramen

(*answers overleaf*)

1.54 **B E**

1.55 **A C D E**
The amnion is *not* a secretory membrane, and amniotic fluid is probably a transudate, with the addition of fetal urine and lung fluid in the second half of pregnancy.

1.56 **A B C D**
Amniotic fluid is only *bacteriostatic* (i.e. inhibits the growth of bacteria), and not bacteriocidal (i.e. capable of killing them).

1.57 **A B D**
The two ventricles do not communicate in the normal fetal circulation, and the ductus arteriosus connects the pulmonary *artery* with the aorta.

1.58 **A B C D E**

1.59 **A D E**
Each innominate bone consists of the ilium, the ischium and the pubis, and the symphysis is not a true synovial joint, but only a pad of fibro-cartilage.

1.60 In the gynaecoid pelvis:
- **A** the brim is triangular and narrowest anteriorly
- **B** the brim is oval, with the widest diameter in the transverse
- **C** it is well shaped for child bearing
- **D** the ischial spines are prominent
- **E** the sacrum is well curved

1.61 A spontaneous 'face-to-pubes' delivery is most likely to occur with which of the following pelvic types?
- **A** android
- **B** osteomalacic
- **C** platypelloid
- **D** anthropoid
- **E** rachitic

1.62 A justo-minor pelvis:
- **A** is caused by trauma
- **B** has both sacral alae missing
- **C** is a generally small, but normally shaped pelvis
- **D** is produced by osteomalacia
- **E** may necessitate operative delivery

1.63 The levator ani muscles:
- **A** constitute the major part of the pelvic floor
- **B** are attached to the pelvic brim
- **C** have fibres inserting into the sacrum and coccyx
- **D** form the apex of the perineal body
- **E** assist defaecation and micturition

1.64 Which of the following muscles constitute the levator ani muscles:
- **A** bulbocavernosus
- **B** iliococcygeus
- **C** ischiocavernosus
- **D** pubococcygeus
- **E** ischiococcygeus

1.65 Which of the following muscles insert into each other in the midline between the vagina and the rectum and anus:
- **A** pubococcygeus
- **B** ischiococcygeus
- **C** transverse perineal muscles
- **D** ischiocavernosus
- **E** bulbocavernosus

(*answers overleaf*)

1.60 **B C E**
A triangular brim and prominent ischial spines are features of an android (male type), pelvis, which is generally unfavourable for childbearing.

1.61 **D**
Because the anthropoid pelvis is usually a roomy pelvis with the widest diameters of both brim and outlet in the antero-posterior.

1.62 **C E**
This is a generally small pelvis, where the reduced diameters may lead to cephalopelvic disproportion and the need for operative or instrumental delivery, unless the fetus is also small.

1.63 **A C D E**

1.64 **B D E**

1.65 **A C**
This is an important point when prolonged distension of the perineal area occurs during labour. These muscle fibres, inserted into each other, can part company when overstretched, and may never regain their elasticity, so impairing the whole integrity of the pelvic floor.

1.66 The perineal body is a pyramid-shaped wedge of muscle and fibrous tissue, and contains fibres from the following pelvic floor muscles:
- **A** external anal sphincter
- **B** transverse perineal muscles
- **C** bulbocavernosus
- **D** pubococcygeus
- **E** iliococcygeus

1.67 The hormones produced by the corpus luteum are:
- **A** oestrogen
- **B** progesterone
- **C** chorionic gonadotrophin
- **D** follicle stimulating hormone
- **E** luteinising hormone

1.68 Human chorionic gonadotrophin:
- **A** is produced by the decidua
- **B** has a similar action to oxytocin
- **C** is excreted in the urine in increasing quantities during late pregnancy
- **D** is secreted by the trophoblast
- **E** produces a positive pregnancy test

1.69 The pituitary gland:
- **A** is situated in the deep fossa in the sphenoid bone
- **B** produces follicle stimulating and luteinising hormones
- **C** has a direct functional link with the hypothalamus
- **D** is an endocrine gland
- **E** produces oxytocin

1.70 Menstruation is the result of:
- **A** failure of the corpus luteum
- **B** high levels of luteinising hormone
- **C** follicle stimulating hormone
- **D** a fall in the progesterone level
- **E** a rise in the level of oestrogens

1.71 The ureters:
- **A** measure approximately 25 cm (10 in) in length
- **B** cross the pelvic brim, close to the sacro-iliac joint, before entering the bladder
- **C** are lined with ciliated epithelium
- **D** pass through the inguinal canal
- **E** lie outside the peritoneal cavity

(*answers overleaf*)

1.66 **A B C D**

1.67 **A B**

1.68 **D E**
Chorionic gonadotrophin is the basis of all pregnancy tests, and must therefore be produced by *fetal* tissue. It is excreted in the maternal urine in large amounts in early pregnancy, but decreases markedly in the latter half of pregnancy.

1.69 **A B C D E**

1.70 **A D**
When the function of the corpus luteum declines, approximately 12–14 days after ovulation, oestrogen and progesterone levels fall quickly, causing the vascular secretory endometrium to be shed as menstrual flow.

1.71 **A B E**
The ureters are lined with transitional epithelium.

1.72 The bregma:

A has three suture lines running into it
B closes after about 18 months
C is the posterior fontanelle
D closes soon after birth
E is diamond shaped

1.73 The normal position of the non-pregnant uterus is:

A anteversion
B retroversion
C hyperextension
D anteflexion
E retroflexion

(*answers overleaf*)

1.72 **B E**

The bregma is the *anterior* fontanelle and has *four* suture lines running into it.

1.73 **A D**

The normal anteverted position of the uterus is assisted by the supporting action of the utero-sacral ligaments posteriorly, and the round ligaments anteriorly.

SECTION III
Questions 1.74–1.81

1.74 Figure 1

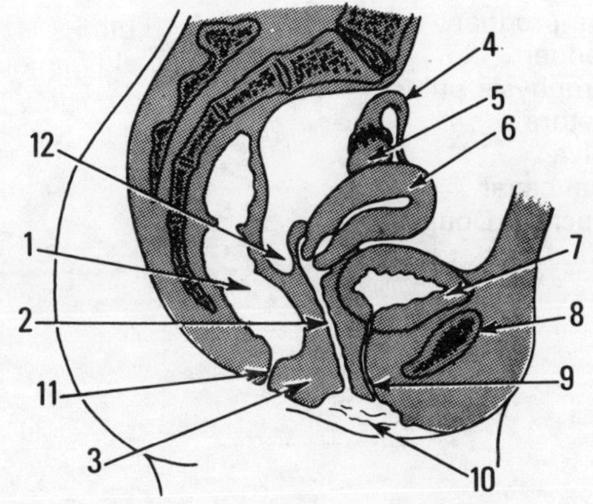

Label this diagram showing a sagittal section through a female pelvis and its contents.

1.75 Figure 2

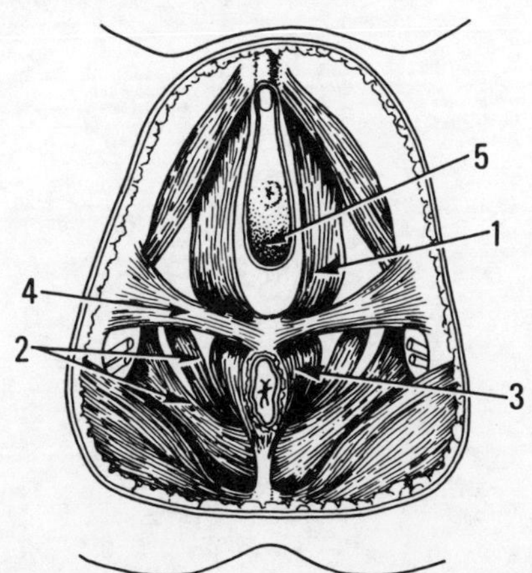

From the items listed below label the diagram correctly:

A clitoris
B transverse perineal muscle
C external anal sphincter
D levator ani muscle
E vagina
F ischiocavernosus
G bulbocavernosus

(*answers overleaf*)

1.74
1 Rectum
2 Vagina
3 Perineal body
4 Uterine (Fallopian) tube
5 Ovary
6 Non-pregnant uterus
7 Bladder
8 Symphysis pubis
9 Urethra
10 Vulva
11 Anal canal
12 Pouch of Douglas

1.75
1 **G**
2 **D**
3 **C**
3 **B**
5 **E**

1.76 Figure 3

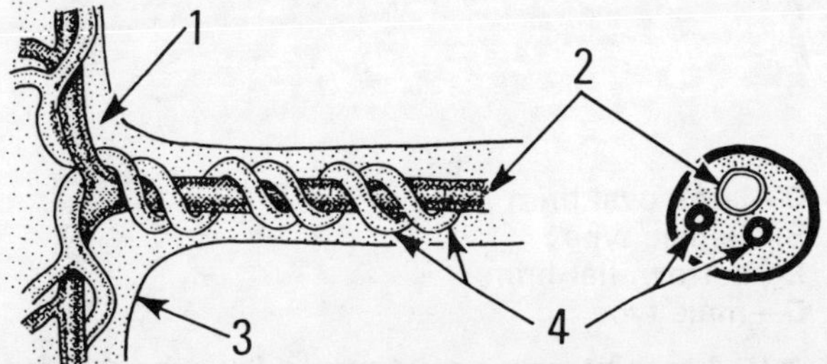

The diagrams above represent the umbilical cord. Match each numbered structure with the appropriate answer from the list given below:

- **A** umbilical vein
- **B** umbilical arteries
- **C** Wharton's jelly
- **D** chorionic villi
- **E** chorion
- **F** amnion
- **G** vasa praevia

1.77 Figure 4

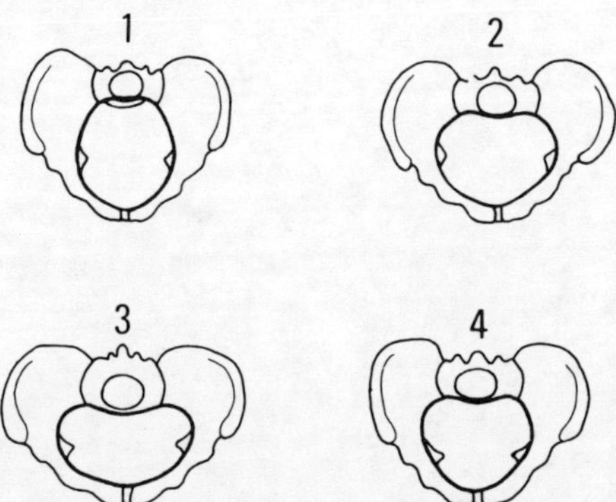

The diagrams show four naturally occurring pelvic types. Match each with its correct name from the list below:

- **A** rachitic
- **B** gynaecoid
- **C** anthropoid
- **D** android
- **E** platypelloid

(*answers overleaf*)

1.76

1 **C**
2 **A**
3 **F**
4 **B**

1.77

1 **C**—large oval brim
2 **B**—female type
3 **E**—narrow, flat brim
4 **D**—male type

N.B. A rachitic pelvis may have a flat brim, but is the product of disease (rickets).

1.78 Figure 5

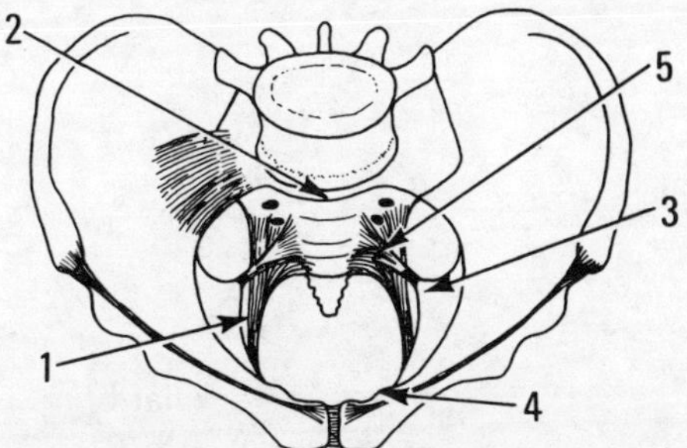

Match each numbered structure shown on the diagram with the appropriate item from the list below:

A sacro-iliac joint
B sacrospinous ligament
C sacrotuberous ligament
D iliopectineal eminence
E sacral promontory
F ischial spine
G pubic tubercle

1.79 Figure 6

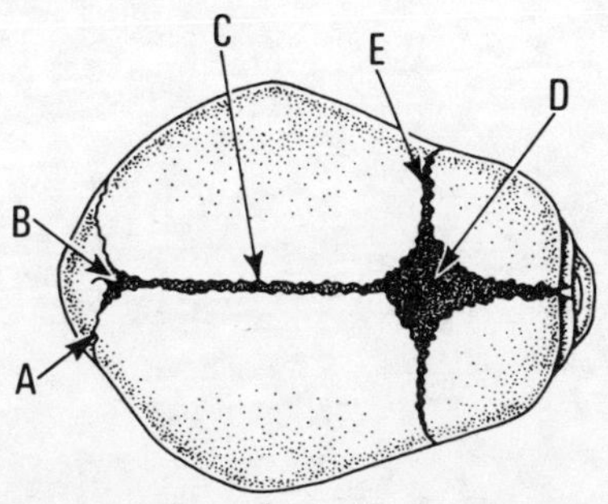

This diagram shows the fetal skull:

1 Which label refers to the fontanelle which closes at 18 months?
2 Which label indicates the bregma?
3 Which label indicates the posterior fontanelle?
4 Which label indicates the suture that is most easily felt on vaginal examination?
5 Which label indicates the lambda?
6 Which label indicates the lambdoid suture?
7 Which label indicates the coronal suture?
8 Which label indicates the sagittal suture?

(*answers overleaf*)

1.78

1 **C**
2 **E**
3 **F**
4 **G**
5 **B**

1.79

1 **D**
2 **D**
3 **B**
4 **C**
5 **B**
6 **A**
7 **E**
8 **C**

1.80 Figure 7

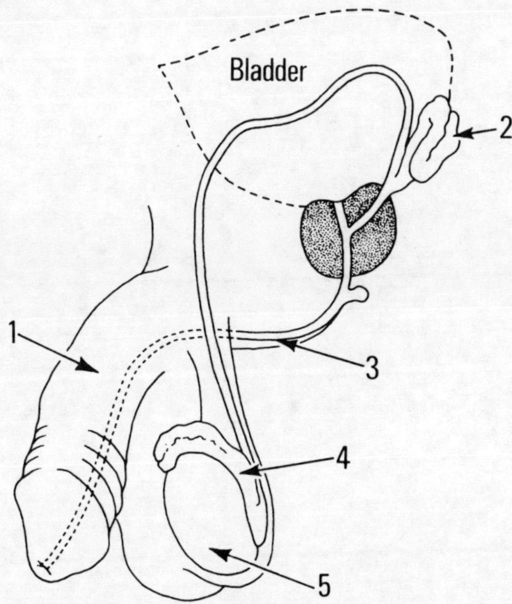

Male reproductive organs. Match each numbered structure shown on the diagram with the appropriate item from the list below:

A urethra
B penis
C testis
D seminal vesicles
E prostate gland
F epididymis

(*answers overleaf*)

1.80

1 **B**
2 **D**
3 **A**
4 **F**
5 **C**

1.81 Figure 8

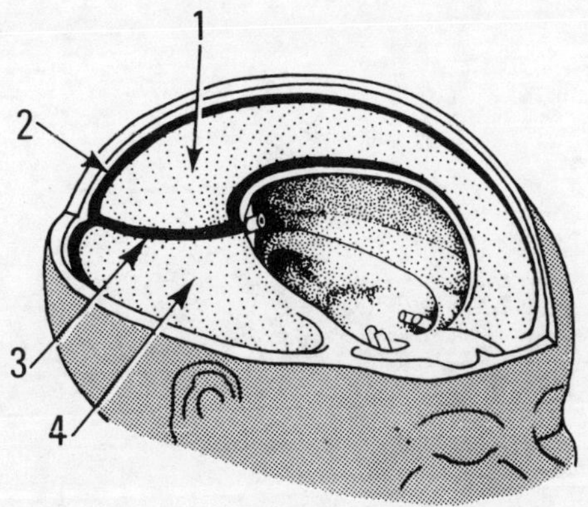

Open Skull—showing skull membranes. Match each numbered structure shown on the diagram with the appropriate item from the list below:

- **A** superior longitudinal sinus
- **B** straight sinus
- **C** falx cerebri
- **D** tentorium cerebelli
- **E** lateral sinus
- **F** circle of Willis

(*answers overleaf*)

1.81

1 **C**
2 **A**
3 **B**
4 **D**

SECTION IV
TRUE OR FALSE? Questions 1.82–1.96

Indicate whether you think the statements listed below are 'true' or 'false'.

Example: **The epiglottis covers the larynx (glottis), and vocal cords, and has to be moved aside when endotracheal intubation is attempted.**

Answer: **True**

1.82 **At the pelvic brim in a gynaecoid pelvis the transverse diameter is the greatest.**

1.83 **At the pelvic outlet in a gynaecoid pelvis the transverse diameter is the greatest.**

1.84 **The sub-pubic arch has an angle of less than 90° in a gynaecoid pelvis.**

1.85 **The antero-posterior diameter of the outlet is measured between the coccyx and the inferior border of the symphysis pubis.**

1.86 **The antero-posterior diameter is the largest at the brim of an anthropoid pelvis.**

1.87 **Oxytocin stimulates breast milk production.**

1.88 **Bartholin's glands lie on either side of the urethral orifice at the vulva.**

1.89 **Vaginal acidity is caused by the lactic acid produced by Döderlein's bacilli.**

1.90 **Overstretching of the pelvic floor may lead to uterine prolapse in later life.**

1.91 **Skene's ducts can be damaged, if an episiotomy is lateral rather than *medio*-lateral.**

1.92 **A third degree laceration, if not correctly repaired, can lead to a recto-vaginal fistula.**

1.93 **In labour, the pelvic floor directs the leading part of the fetus forward to lie under the symphysis pubis.**

(*answers overleaf*)

1.82 **True**

1.83 **False**
The antero-posterior diameter of the outlet is the greatest.

1.84 **False**
In a gynaecoid pelvis the sub-pubic angle should measure at least 90°.

1.85 **False**
The antero-posterior diameter of the outlet is measured from the lower border of the sacrum, because the coccyx is mobile and is not a fixed point.

1.86 **True**
This is why the fetus is generally positioned directly occipito-anterior or occipito-posterior, and because the anthropoid pelvis is usually of generous proportions, some occipito-posterior positions will deliver spontaneously face-to-pubes.

1.87 **False**
Prolactin stimulates actual milk production, while oxytocin causes the myo-epithelial cells around the alveoli and duct system to contract, and thus pump milk along to the ampullae and nipple while the baby is suckling.

1.88 **False**
Bartholin's glands are two compound racemose glands which lie on either side of the posterior aspect of the vaginal orifice. They secrete mucus and discharge it into the lower part of the vagina via two narrow ducts. Skene's tubules lie on either side of the lower urethra.

1.89 **True**
Döderlein's bacilli are part of the normal flora of a healthy vagina. They act on the glycogen stored in the cells of the squamous epithelial lining of the vagina to produce lactic acid. The vaginal pH is approximately 4.5 during reproductive life, and this acidity helps to destroy any pathogens which invade the vagina.

1.90 **True**

1.91 **False**
Bartholin's ducts may be damaged by a lateral episiotomy.

1.92 **True**

1.93 **True**

1.94 **The android pelvis is a deep, heavy pelvis, and often has a flat sacrum.**

1.95 **A 'high assimilation' pelvis has a flat, narrow brim.**

1.96 **Anterior asynclitism is where the fetal head is tilted to allow the anterior parietal bone to enter the pelvis first, thus allowing the smallest diameter of the head to pass through the pelvic brim, (i.e. the super-sub-parietal diameter).**

(answers overleaf)

1.94 **True**

1.95 **False**
A high assimilation pelvis is where the 5th lumbar vertebra is fused to the sacrum, so that there are *six* fused vertebrae instead of the usual five. This is most frequently seen in the anthropoid type of pelvis.

1.96 **True**
The super-sub-parietal diameter (8.25 cm approximately) measures considerably less than the bi-parietal diameter (9.5 cm approximately) which generally passes through the pelvic brim.

Figure 9

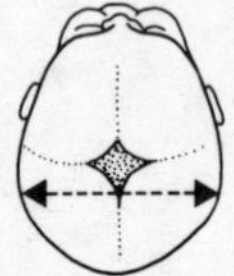

Biparietal diameter

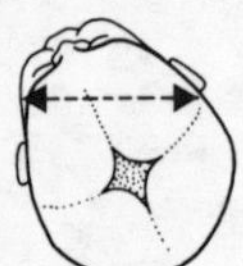

Super-sub-parietal diameter in anterior asynclitism

SECTION V
MATCHING ITEMS Questions 1.97–1.99

Match the items in Group 1 with the most suitable item in Group 2. (Each item in Group 2 may only be used *once.*)

Example: **Match the items in Group 1 with the most suitable item in Group 2:**

Group 1		*Group 2*
(i) anterior fontanelle	**A**	oestrogen production
(ii) ovary	**B**	spermatozoa
(iii) testes	**C**	chorionic gonadotrophin
(iv) vagina	**D**	acid medium
	E	bregma

Answer:

(i) E
(ii) A
(iii) B
(iv) D

1.97 Match the items in Group 1 with the most suitable item in Group 2:

Group 1		*Group 2*
(i) round ligaments	**A**	pelvic floor
(ii) levator ani muscles	**B**	mesosalpinx
(iii) urinary bladder	**C**	Fallopian tube
(iv) ciliated epithelium	**D**	anteversion of the uterus
	E	detrusor muscle

1.98 Match the items in Group 1 with the most suitable item in Group 2:

Group 1		*Group 2*
(i) anterior pituitary gland	**A**	suckling
(ii) development of breast alveoli	**B**	myo-epithelial cells
(iii) oxytocin	**C**	progesterone
(iv) stimulus to lactation	**D**	antidiuretic hormone
	E	luteinising hormone

1.99 Match the items in Group 1 with the most appropriate item in Group 2.

Group 1		*Group 2*
(i) anthropoid pelvis	**A**	spontaneous face-to-pubes delivery
(ii) android pelvis	**B**	missing sacral ala
(iii) platypelloid pelvis	**C**	narrow sub-pubic arch
(iv) gynaecoid pelvis	**D**	flat, kidney-shaped brim
	E	well curved sacrum

(*answers overleaf*)

1.97

(i) **D**
(ii) **A**
(iii) **E**
(iv) **C**

1.98

(i) **E**
(ii) **C**
(iii) **B**
(iv) **A**

1.99

(i) **A**
(ii) **C**
(iii) **D**
(iv) **E**

A missing sacral ala is associated with a rare congenital abnormality known as Naegele's pelvis. When *both* sacral alae are missing it is known as Robert's pelvis.

SECTION VI
ASSERTION/REASON Question 1.100–1.103

Read carefully the 5 possible answers listed below marked A, B, C, D, and E, and select which is appropriate for the assertions and reasons which follow:

A Assertion true, reason is a true statement, and is the *correct* reason.
B Assertion and reason both true, but reason is *not* the correct reason.
C Assertion is true, but reason is a false statement.
D Assertion is false, but the reason is a true statement.
E Assertion and reason are both false.

Example: **The fetal skull can mould during labour**
because
the bones of the vault are laid down in membrane.

Answer: **A** Both the assertion and the reason are correct, and the reason is the correct reason.

1.100 Screening for carcinoma of the cervix can be easily carried out
because
epithelial cells from the squamo-columnar junction can be obtained by a simple test.

1.101 The platypelloid pelvis is unsuited for easy childbearing
because
it has both sacral alae missing.

1.102 In pregnancy the number of red blood cells in the circulation falls
because
there is physiological haemodilution.

1.103 Vulvo-vaginitis is more common in young girls and elderly women
because
the vaginal acidity is increased before puberty and in post-menopausal women.

(*answers overleaf*)

1.100 **A**

1.101 **C**
The platypelloid pelvis has a flat brim which makes it unfavourable for childbearing.
Where *both* sacral alae are absent, it is known as Robert's pelvis.

1.102 **D**
There is an actual increase in red blood cells in pregnancy, but because there is an even larger increase in plasma volume, a physiological haemodilution occurs, and the haemoglobin level actually falls.

1.103 **C**
The acidity of the vagina is markedly reduced in pre-pubertal girls and after the menopause as less Döderlein's bacilli are present. The more alkaline environment encourages the growth of vaginal pathogens such as *Candida albicans*, so that vulvo-vaginitis in the young and senile vaginitis in the elderly is common.

SECTION VII
COMPLETION ITEMS Questions 1.104–1.111

Complete the following sentences with the appropriate word(s).

Example: **The ovarian cortex contains numerous____________which are the functional units of the ovary.**

Answer: Graafian follicles.

1.104 The perineal body derives its blood supply from the ________ artery.

1.105 The____________nerve passes round the ischial spine before it re-enters the pelvis, and supplies the major portion of the pelvic floor.

1.106 During its initial development, the fertilised ovum is called a____________, but by the time it reaches the uterine cavity, it has become a____________, and shows an inner cell mass and an outer trophoblastic layer.

1.107 As the blastocyst begins to develop into an embryo, two small cavities appear in the inner cell mass. These are known as the____________sac and the____________sac.

1.108 Following this, three distinct types of tissue are found, which then form all the body structures. ECTODERM produces outer structures such as____________

____

MESODERM produces midline structures such as____________.

and ENTODERM forms internal structures such as____________.

1.109 The____________is the outer membrane, and is continuous with the placenta. The inner membrane is the ____________and covers the placenta and cord.

1.110 In the second half of the menstrual cycle, the endometrium is described as____________, and at this time it is extremely vascular and secretes____________, to nourish a possible fertilised ovum.

(*answers overleaf*)

1.104 Internal pudendal artery

1.105 Pudendal nerve

1.106 a Morula
b Blastocyst

1.107 a Yolk sac
b Amniotic sac

1.108 a (Ectoderm) skin; nails; lens of the eye; enamel of the teeth, and even the central nervous system, as in early embryonic development the nervous system is an external structure until the skull bones and vertebral column surround it for protection.
b (Mesoderm) the heart; blood; blood vessels; lymphatics; bones; muscles; kidneys; gonads.
c (Entoderm) alimentary tract; liver; pancreas; lungs; thyroid gland.

1.109 a Chorion
b Amnion

1.110 a Secretory
b Glycogen

1.111 **The lambdoidal sutures separate the____________________ and the ____________________bones, and where they are joined by the____________________suture form the____________________fontanelle, which closes at approximately____________________after birth.**

(*answers overleaf*)

1.111

a Occiput
b Parietal bones
c Sagittal
d Posterior fontanelle (or lambda)
e Six weeks

ANATOMY AND PHYSIOLOGY

The following questions are taken from recent examination papers set by the English National Board.

1. Essay questions (*These questions are allocated 45 minutes*)

Describe the anatomy and functions of the placenta. Discuss how placental function may be monitored in pregnancy. (1983)

Describe the physiology of micturition and the possible disturbances of micturition which may occur in the postnatal period. (1983)

Describe the perineal body. Discuss the effects of perineal discomfort on a woman in the puerperium, and the possible managment by a midwife. (1983)

Describe how minor disorders relate to the physiological changes of pregnancy. (1983)

Describe the anatomy of the pelvic floor. How may a midwife reduce the risk of damage to this structure? (1983)

Describe the physiology of lactation. Discuss the possible problems encountered by a mother who is breast feeding her baby. (1983)

Describe the physiology of the third stage of labour. Outline *TWO* methods by which a midwife may manage this stage of labour. (1983)

Describe the fetal skull. How may this knowledge be applied during the managment of labour? (1983)

Describe the physiological changes which occur in a mother during the puerperium. How does the midwife assess that these changes are taking place? (1983)

Outline the functions of the placenta. Explain how fetal well-being may be assessed during pregnancy. (1984)

Outline the changes which occur in the uterus during pregnancy. What factors influence variation in uterine size during the latter half of pregnancy? (1984)

Describe the physiological changes in the urinary tract during pregnancy. Discuss the significance of abnormal constituents which may be found on urinalysis. (1984)

**Outline the physiological changes occurring in the second stage of labour.
Discuss the midwife's role during this stage. (1984)**

**Describe the anatomy of the breasts.
Mrs Dawkins, a primigravida, wishes to breast feed her baby. How would you meet her needs in this respect throughout pregnancy? (1984)**

**Describe the normal physiological changes which occur in the fetus during labour and the birth process, which assist the baby to adapt to its new environment.
How would you monitor these changes? (1984)**

**How may a knowledge of amniotic fluid be used in the diagnosis of complications during pregnancy?
When an amniocentesis is being considered, what factors should the midwife discuss with the prospective parents? (1984)**

**What is the composition of human breast milk?
How should cow's milk be modified to make it suitable for the neonate? (1984)**

Describe the vault of the fetal skull including the internal anatomy. How may this knowledge assist the midwife in her care of a woman during labour? (1984)

Describe the anatomy of the breasts and the physiology of lactation. Why may a mother fail to breast feed her baby successfully? (1984)

Describe the size, shape and landmarks of the gynaecoid pelvis. How would you use your knowledge of the pelvis in the management of pregnancy?

**What changes in maternal physiology can give rise to the minor disorders of pregnancy?
What advice and support can a midwife give to alleviate these disorders? (1985)**

**Pelvic floor damage may impair a woman's health.
Describe the anatomy of the pelvic floor.
How may a midwife prevent or minimise pelvic floor damage? (1985)**

2. Write briefly on each of the following subjects (these short questions are allocated 7–10 minutes each):

Blastocyst (1983)
Physiology of lactation (1983)
Lochia (1983)
Influence of an anthropoid pelvis on labour (1983)
Anterior fontanelle (1983)
Amniotic fluid (1983)
Production of spermatozoa (1984)

The skin of the neonate (1984)
Initiation of lactation (1984)
Oestriol in pregnancy (1984)
Meconium (1984)
The cervix (1984)
Succenturiate placenta (1984)
The pelvic outlet (1984)
Moulding of the fetal skull (1984)
Human chorionic gonadotrophin (1985)
Normal uterine action (1985)

2. Pregnancy

SECTION I
Questions 2.1–2.25

Select a *single* correct response to each of the following questions:

2.1 The commonest cause of amenorrhoea is:
A metropathia
B menorrhagia
C salpingitis
D pregnancy

2.2 Human chorionic gonadotrophin is found in the:
A urine during pregnancy
B blood at all times
C cervical mucus
D menstrual flow

2.3 In pregnancy the muscle fibres of the uterus increase in size by a process of:
A hypertrophy
B hypertrophy and hyperplasia
C hyperplasia and autolysis
D aplasia

2.4 In a normal pregnancy total weight gain should not exceed:
A 5 kg
B 9 kg
C 13 kg
D 17 kg

(*answers overleaf*)

2.1 **D**

Metropathia haemorrhagica is a disorder of menstruation characterised by irregular and/or heavy bleeding. Menorrhagia is *excessive* menstrual loss.

2.2 **A**

The detection of chorionic gonadotrophin in the urine forms the basis for pregnancy testing.

2.3 **B**

Existing muscle fibres enlarge (hypertrophy), but new fibres are also laid down (hyperplasia).

2.4 **C**

11–13 kg can be taken as a guide to average total weight gain in pregnancy.

2.5 The pregnant uterus does not normally reach the level of the xiphisternum until:

A 38 weeks
B 36 weeks
C 34 weeks
D 32 weeks

2.6 Routine antenatal blood tests include estimation of maternal antibodies to:

A German measles
B measles
C whooping cough
D chicken pox

2.7 The earliest stage of pregnancy at which a multipara notices quickening is:

A 12 weeks
B 16 weeks
C 20 weeks
D 24 weeks

2.8 The lie of the fetus *in utero*, is the relationship of:

A the long axis of the fetus to the mother's pelvis
B the denominator to the mother's pelvis
C the attitude of the fetus to the uterus
D the long axis of the fetus to the long axis of the uterus

2.9 If, on abdominal examination, the uterus appears small for the duration of amenorrhoea, this may be due to:

A intra-uterine growth retardation
B the presence of fibroids in the uterus
C multiple pregnancy
D polyhydramnios

2.10 A pregnant woman who has a history of one normal confinement, and one unexplained stillbirth:

A may properly be booked for home confinement
B may properly be booked for a general practitioner unit
C should not have a vaginal examination until 16 weeks' gestation
D requires a screening test for syphilis, even though it was previously negative

2.11 Heavy smoking during pregnancy predisposes the infant to:

A spina bifida
B respiratory distress syndrome
C atelectasis.
D low birth weight

(*answers overleaf*)

2.5 **B**

2.6 **A**
The majority of women now have a screening test for rubella antibodies carried out at the 'booking' visit.

2.7 **B**
Occasionally a woman may say she has felt movements earlier than this, but is uncommon, and should make one wonder if her expected date of delivery has been calculated correctly.

2.8 **D**

2.9 **A**
Multiple pregnancy, fibroids and polyhydramnios would all make the uterus appear *large*-for-dates.

2.10 **D**
Unexplained stillbirths mean that the patient should be seen by a consultant obstetrician throughout pregnancy, and delivered in a consultant unit. As syphilis can be a cause of stillbirth, the screening tests should definitely be repeated for every pregnancy.

2.11 **D**
There is now clear evidence that heavy smoking during pregnancy can cause both pre-term labour and low birth weight babies.

2.12 Vaginal bleeding before the 28th week of pregnancy is termed:
A threatened abortion
B carneous mole
C antepartum haemorrhage
D hydatidiform mole

2.13 Which of the following equates with 8 stone 4 lb:
A 52.5 kg
B 57.0 kg
C 59.5 kg
D 62.0 kg

2.14 Which of the following symbols may be used to indicate micrograms?
A mgm
B mg
C ml
D μg

2.15 Imperfect fusion of the two Müllerian ducts in early intrauterine life, can lead to:
A retroverted uterus
B double uterus
C intramural fibroids
D ovarian cyst

2.16 The most *serious* sign of pre-eclampsia is:
A excessive weight gain
B proteinuria
C occult oedema
D hypertension

2.17 The red blood cells in folic acid deficiency anaemia are described as:
A microcytic
B megaloblastic
C hypochromic
D polymorphic

2.18 Anterior obliquity is a:
A cystocele
B asynclitism
C pendulous abdomen
D bicornuate uterus

(*answers overleaf*)

2.12 **A**

Obviously threatened abortion can be due to a hydatidiform mole or a carneous mole, although frank bleeding is not a *marked* feature of either condition. Vaginal bleeding later than the 28th week is termed antepartum haemorrhage.

2.13 **A**

1 kg = 2.2 lb

2.14 **D**

However, it is much safer actually to write the term 'microgram' out in full, than to use the symbol 'μg'

2.15 **B**

There are various manifestations of this problem, which can cause considerable gynaecological and obstetric problems, and other examples include double vagina, sub-septate uterus etc.

2.16 **B**

Significant proteinuria indicates renal involvement, and is always a serious sign. It generally means that the disease is worsening, despite conservative treatment.

2.17 **B**

Folic acid deficiency produces a megaloblastic anaemia, where the red cells are larger than normal, and in an immature stage of development. In pregnancy it can be associated with multiple pregnancy, or (more rarely, in this country,) dietary deficiency. In iron-deficiency anaemia, the red blood cells are described as microcytic (small) and hypochromic (pale), the latter being due to the lack of haemoglobin.

2.18 **C**

This can be an extremely uncomfortable condition in multiparous women who have very poor abdominal wall muscles. Malpresentations may be associated with this condition, and some form of corset is required to support the growing uterus.

2.19 Placenta praevia is:

A vasa praevia
B placental abruption
C a normally sited placenta
D an abnormally sited placenta

(*answers overleaf*)

2.19 **D**

A placenta praevia is *abnormally* sited as it wholly or partly occupies the lower uterine segment. Placental abruption (abruptio placentae) is when there is premature separation and bleeding from a *normally* sited placenta (i.e. in the upper segment). Vasa praevia may occur with a velamentous insertion of cord, when the unprotected blood vessels running in the membranes lie *in front of the presenting part.* These vessels are very prone to damage when the membranes rupture, and lethal fetal haemorrhage can occur.

Figure 10

Velamentous insertion of cord

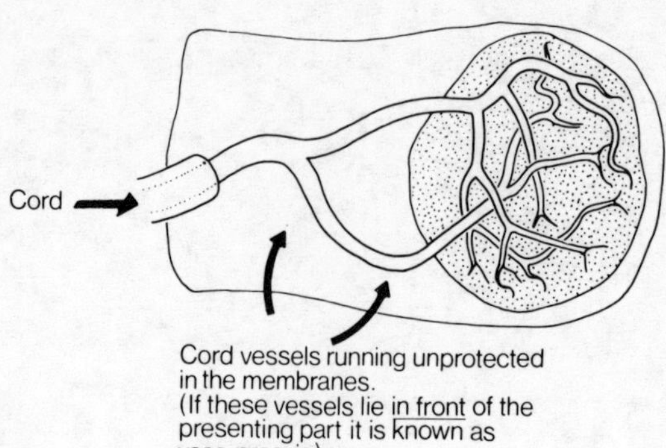

CASE HISTORY

A primigravida presents with mild, painless, bleeding per vaginam at 35 weeks of pregnancy. Following admission and two days of complete bedrest, a further more severe episode of painless bleeding occurs. Apart from an easily felt breech presentation, no other abnormalities are discovered.

The following six questions relate to the above history.

2.20 The probable diagnosis is:
A placental abruption
B accidental antepartum haemorrhage
C placenta praevia
D cervical erosion

2.21 An ultrasound scan may be carried out to:
A exclude cord prolapse
B estimate liquor volume
C detect any fetal abnormality
D localise the placenta

2.22 Because of the risk of further haemorrhage it is important to:
A give a fibrinogen infusion
B cross match blood
C give parenteral iron therapy
D estimate the haemoglobin level daily

2.23 In order to exclude incidental haemorrhage the obstetrician may perform a:
A vaginal examination
B pelvic examination
C speculum examination
D abdominal examination

2.24 If it appears necessary to expedite delivery, amniocentesis may be performed to estimate:
A Pea-Wea score
B liquor volume
C vernix content
D lecithin-sphingomyelin ratio

2.25 The most likely mode of delivery will be:
A caesarean section
B ventouse extraction
C spontaneous vaginal delivery
D Kielland's forceps delivery

(*answers overleaf*)

2.20 **C**

2.21 **D**

2.22 **B**

2.23 **C**

2.24 **D**

This is to gauge fetal lung maturity. If the lecithin-sphingomyelin ratio is less than 2:1, it may be appropriate to give the mother a steroid preparation such as betamethazone in an attempt to stimulate surfactant production in the fetus, although some authorities feel there is now evidence that this may have undesirable sequelae for the fetus.

The Pea-Wea score is used to assess the fetal condition prenatally. It is based on estimations of fetal heart rate patterns in response to fetal activity and uterine contractions.

2.25 **A**

Except in very minor degrees of placenta praevia, the fetus will be delivered by elective caesarean section, to minimise maternal blood loss and safeguard the fetus.

SECTION II
MULTIPLE RESPONSE QUESTIONS Questions 2.26–2.60

Select any number of correct responses between 1–5.

2.26 Which of the following are normal symptoms of pregnancy in the first trimester:
A dyspnoea
B fetal movement
C nausea and vomiting
D heartburn
E frequency of micturition

2.27 Proteinuria may be an indication of:
A urinary tract infection
B phenylketonuria
C diabetes mellitus
D adrenal tumours
E pre-eclampsia

2.28 Pregnancy can be *positively* diagnosed in the presence of:
A striae gravidarum
B progressive enlargement of the uterus
C amenorrhoea
D audible fetal heart sounds
E palpation of fetal parts

2.29 The physiological increase in blood volume in pregnancy produces:
A decrease in haemoglobin level
B reduction in platelet count
C increased cardiac output
D reduction in leucocyte count
E increased weight gain

2.30 Which of the following groups of patients has a high priority for confinement in a consultant unit:
A mothers in their second or third pregnancy
B previous postpartum haemorrhage
C a history of low birth weight babies
D multigravid patients under 30 years of age
E unsuitable home conditions

(*answers overleaf*)

2.26 **C E**
'Quickening', heartburn and dyspnoea tend to occur in the 2nd or 3rd trimester.

2.27 **A E**

2.28 **D E**
Amenorrhoea, striae gravidarum, and uterine enlargement are probable, but not *positive* signs of pregnancy.

2.29 **A C E**
The increased blood volume consists of a significantly larger rise in plasma volume than red cells, hence the physiological fall in the haemoglobin level. The increased volume raises the cardiac output, and also accounts for some weight gain. Platelet and white cell counts usually *rise* during pregnancy.

2.30 **B C**
Multigravid patients under 30, having their second or third child, with no other complications, could reasonably be booked for a general practitioner unit or even a home confinement if they so wished. Patients with unsuitable home conditions could be confined in *either* a consultant or general practitioner unit.

2.31 Bleeding per vaginam in early pregnancy could be due to:
A tubal pregnancy
B accidental antepartum haemorrhage
C threatened abortion
D cervical polyp
E haemorrhoids

2.32 If the mother contracts rubella in early pregnancy, when organogenesis is in progress, the following defects can occur in the fetus:
A cardiac abnormalities
B cataracts
C talipes
D microcephaly
E extra digit

2.33 Testing the mother's blood at about 17–18 weeks of pregnancy for alpha-feto-protein, may help to diagnose:
A microcephaly
B open neural tube defects
C myelomeningocele
D syphilis
E anencephaly

2.34 Grande multiparity:
A is characterised by prolonged labour
B has an increased maternal mortality and morbidity rate
C is frequently associated with anaemia
D is most harmful in Social Classes IV and V
E usually denotes four or more past pregnancies

2.35 Polyhydramnios may be associated with:
A diabetes mellitus
B heartburn and dyspnoea
C a fluid 'thrill'
D unstable lie
E malpresentation

2.36 External cephalic version is not favoured by all obstetricians, and is definitely contra-indicated in:
A severe pre-eclampsia
B oligohydramnios
C iron deficiency anaemia
D rhesus iso-immunisation
E twin pregnancy

(*answers overleaf*)

2.31 **A C D**
Antepartum haemorrhage by definition occurs *after* 28 weeks of pregnancy, which cannot be classified as *early* pregnancy.

2.32 **A B D**
Deafness may also be a serious handicap.

2.33 **B C E**
This test, if positive, may indicate some form of open neural tube defect, and should be confirmed by amniocentesis. A *slightly* raised result may be due to multiple pregnancy.

2.34 **B C D**
Grande multiparity (having borne 4 or more *children*) is often associated with very rapid labours and other problems such as unstable lie, and postpartum haemorrhage. In Social Classes IV and V, lower intelligence and financial constraints may lead to poorly-spaced pregnancies, poor nutrition and housing, and a low uptake of prenatal care.

2.35 **A B C D E**

2.36 **A B D E**
In severe pre-eclampsia the fetus is already at risk, and version may be the final insult. With a markedly reduced amount of liquor it is usually unsuccessful, and where rhesus antibodies have already been detected, there would be a risk of increasing the antibody titre, should any placental separation occur during the procedure. It is generally considered to be difficult and hazardous to attempt to turn *one* fetus in a multiple pregnancy.

2.37 Asymptomatic bacteriuria:
- **A** is characterised by dysuria
- **B** is present in approximately 5 per cent of pregnant women
- **C** predisposes to pyelonephritis
- **D** occurs only in multiparous women
- **E** often causes abdominal or loin pain

2.38 Pre-eclampsia is characterised by:
- **A** hypertension
- **B** ketonuria
- **C** oedema
- **D** excessive weight gain
- **E** tachypnoea

2.39 During pregnancy, the severity of rhesus disease can be assessed by estimating:
- **A** the number of fetal cells in maternal blood
- **B** the maternal haemoglobin level
- **C** urinary oestriol excretion
- **D** the maternal blood antibody titre
- **E** bile pigment content of liquor following amniocentesis

2.40 Select correct statements on rhesus iso-immunisation:
- **A** The administration of anti-D immunoglobulin to the rhesus negative mother after every pregnancy, will almost always prevent the formation of antibodies.
- **B** Giving anti-D to the baby may prevent haemolytic disease.
- **C** Anti-D need not be given if the father is rhesus positive (heterozygous).
- **D** Amniocentesis may cause a feto-maternal haemorrhage.
- **E** Where no antibodies are present at the first prenatal visit, the rhesus negative woman should be tested again later in pregnancy.

2.41 Placental insufficiency:
- **A** accompanies severe pre-eclampsia
- **B** is frequently associated with maternal anaemia
- **C** often results in low birth weight babies
- **D** usually carries a marked increase in amniotic fluid volume
- **E** is confirmed by estimating the lecithin-sphingomyelin ratio

2.42 Eclampsia may be characterised by:
- **A** epileptiform fits
- **B** supra-pubic pain
- **C** proteinuria
- **D** nausea or vomiting
- **E** glycosuria

(*answers overleaf*)

2.37 **B C**
Asymptomatic bacteriuria has none of the usual clinical signs of urinary tract infection, but laboratory cultures show that the urine contains more than 100 000 organisms per millilitre. If this condition is untreated, then more serious clinical infections may occur, and can become chronic.

2.38 **A C D**
In addition, proteinuria may occur in more serious cases.

2.39 **D E**
The maternal rhesus antibody titre, and the amount of bile pigment detected in the liquor by spectrophotometry, accurately reflect how severely the fetus is affected. This is helpful in planning the management of the pregnancy, and increases the chances of obtaining a live baby.

2.40 **A D E**
Amniocentesis should always be carried out under ultrasound control, so that the placenta can be localised and avoided by the operator.

2.41 **A C**

2.42 **A C D**
Also visual disturbances and epigastric pain. Many of these signs and symptoms may be caused by the widespread oedema, which includes the brain and liver.

2.43 Hyperemesis gravidarum may lead to:
- **A** oliguria
- **B** dehydration
- **C** ketosis
- **D** jaundice
- **E** death

2.44 Acute pyelonephritis in pregnancy:
- **A** may simulate premature labour
- **B** is characterised by loin pain
- **C** is generally caused by Staphylococcus aureus
- **D** has an increased incidence in pre-eclampsia
- **E** can simulate concealed antepartum haemorrhage

2.45 Diabetes in pregnancy increases the incidence of:
- **A** pre-eclampsia
- **B** polyhydramnios
- **C** folate deficiency
- **D** excessively large babies
- **E** congenital abnormalities

2.46 Which of the following conditions predispose to hypofibrinogenaemia?
- **A** thalassaemia major
- **B** placenta praevia
- **C** intra-uterine death
- **D** placental abruption
- **E** hyperemesis gravidarum

2.47 Placental function can be monitored by:
- **A** lecithin-sphingomyelin ratios
- **B** serial urinary oestriol assays
- **C** serial bi-parietal cephalometry
- **D** serial human placental lactogen estimations
- **E** antenatal cardiotocography

2.48 In eclampsia, cerebral oedema may occur, and can cause:
- **A** convulsions
- **B** purpura
- **C** frontal headache
- **D** vomiting
- **E** tetany

(*answers overleaf*)

2.43 **A B C D E**
Although severe hyperemesis is not often seen nowadays, if neglected it can lead to serious chloride depletion, electrolyte imbalance, renal and hepatic failure, and even death.

2.44 **A B E**

2.45 **A B D E**

2.46 **C D**
A dead fetus that is not delivered within 2–3 weeks of death, and severe placental abruption, can both lead to a marked decrease in the amount of circulating fibrinogen, and this can lead to torrential haemorrhage in labour.

2.47 **B D**
Bi-parietal cephalometry and cardiotocography are used to assess fetal growth and well-being, but are *not* direct tests of placental function.

2.48 **A C D**

2.49 Which of the following are true statements about breech presentations?

A is always associated with polyhydramnios
B has an incidence in labour of approximately 3 per cent
C may have flexed or extended legs
D engaging diameter is the bi-trochanteric (10 cm)
E has a low perinatal mortality rate

2.50 The effects of diabetes mellitus on pregnancy include an *increased*:

A risk of shoulder dystocia in vaginal delivery
B insulin requirement in the puerperium
C insulin requirement during the pregnancy
D caesarian section rate
E incidence of perinatal death

2.51 The 'elderly' primigravida aged 35 years or more:

A tends to default from prenatal clinics
B has an increased perinatal mortality
C is prone to precipitate delivery
D has an increased incidence of Down's syndrome
E may have reduced fertility

2.52 Oligohydramnios is:

A characterised by a pendulous abdomen
B a rare condition
C caused by an ovarian cyst
D associated with renal agenesis
E usually found with anencephaly

2.53 Amniocentesis may be used to determine:

A fetal maturity
B lecithin-sphingomyelin ratio
C fetal distress
D congenital dislocation of the hip
E bilirubin level

2.54 Anaemia in pregnancy may be due to:

A iron deficiency
B vitamin E deficiency
C diabetes mellitus
D folic acid deficiency
E thalassaemia minor

(*answers overleaf*)

2.49 **B C D**

Breech delivery overall, has an increased perinatal mortality and morbidity.

2.50 **A C D E**

The very large babies born to some diabetics may cause problems with the delivery of impacted shoulders. Insulin requirement in pregnancy is generally increased, and may be difficult to stabilise. In the puerperium however, there is a marked reduction in the need for insulin. The perinatal death rate remains higher than average (10–15 per cent).

2.51 **B D E**

The 'elderly' primigravida is an anxious, *regular* clinic attender, but is more likely to have a longer than average labour, and an increased incidence of operative or instrumental delivery.

2.52 **B D**

True oligohydramnios, where the liquor volume is less than 200–300 ml is rare. There are many pregnancies that have a significant reduction in liquor volume, especially near to term, but few are really oligohydramnios. In the genuine cases, congenital absence of kidneys (renal agenesis) or severe bilateral polycystic kidneys, is a common feature, and can account for the loss of liquor volume, as no fetal urine is produced.

2.53 **A B E**

Liquor may be treated with nile blue sulphate, which will stain the fetal cells orange. The number of fetal cells shed into the liquor increases in late pregnancy, and can be a helpful guide to maturity.

2.54 **A D E**

Thalassaemia minor is a condition seen mainly in people with origins in the Mediterranean regions. The haemoglobin is abnormal, (haemoglobinopathy), and red cell survival is reduced. Excessive iron therapy is *contra-indicated* as the patient cannot utilise extra iron.

2.55 The following drugs are anti-hypertensive agents:

A guanethidine (Ismelin)
B bethanidine (Esbatal)
C vitamin K_1 (Konakion)
D ergometrine maleate
E hydrallazine (Apresoline)

2.56 The most common cardiac lesions seen in pregnancy are:

A aortic incompetence
B mitral stenosis
C septal defects
D Fallot's tetralogy
E coarctation of the aorta

2.57 The woman with a moderate to severe cardiac lesion is most at risk during:

A 12th–16th weeks of pregnancy
B 28th–34th weeks of pregnancy
C first stage of labour
D second stage of labour
E third stage of labour

(*answers overleaf*)

2.55 **A B E**
Ergometrine has a tendency to *raise the blood pressure.*

2.56 **A B C**
Rheumatic disease of mitral and aortic valves is still the commonest type of heart disease encountered in pregnancy. However, the improvement in cardiac surgery has meant more children with cardiac defects survive to adulthood and bear their own offspring.

2.57 **B E**
Between the 28th–34th weeks of pregnancy, the blood volume, and thus the cardiac output, reaches its maximum. Also, during the third stage of labour, following placental separation, at least 500–600 ml blood is shunted back into the systemic circulation from the placental bed, and at both these times the mother may easily go into cardiac failure, and even die.

CASE HISTORY 1

A young primigravida is admitted as an emergency at 11 weeks' gestation, with acute lower abdominal pain and retention of urine.

Using the above information, answer the following three questions:

2.58 The possible diagnoses are:
- **A** acute pyelonephritis
- **B** incarcerated, retroverted gravid uterus
- **C** spontaneous pneumothorax
- **D** cholecystitis
- **E** premature labour

2.59 When a retroverted uterus becomes incarcerated in the sacral hollow in early pregnancy, the bladder may become grossly distended with several litres of urine. It is important that the bladder is emptied:
- **A** by self-retaining catheter
- **B** slowly
- **C** by supra-pubic aspiration
- **D** quickly
- **E** by stimulating the bladder to contract with a drug such as Carbachol

2.60 The dangers of this condition if neglected are:
- **A** incompetent cervix
- **B** dextrorotation of the uterus
- **C** spontaneous abortion
- **D** rupture of the bladder
- **E** rectocele

(*answers overleaf*)

2.58 **A B**

2.59 **A B**

The bladder must be drained *slowly* to minimise the risk of abortion. Drugs such as Carbachol should *never* be used in these circumstances.

2.60 **C D**

CASE HISTORY 2

Annette is a 26-year-old and has an active toddler—Kevin, aged 2. She is now pregnant for the second time, and on a routine visit to her antenatal clinic at 34 weeks gestation her midwife and obstetrician both agree that her uterus is significantly smaller than expected for the estimated period of pregnancy.

With reference to the above information answer the questions which follow:

2.61 The most accurate estimation of duration of pregnancy can be achieved by:
- **A** ultrasound scanning in the first trimester
- **B** serial human placental lactogen levels
- **C** estimation of human chorionic gonadotrophin levels
- **D** serial ultrasound scans in the last trimester
- **E** abdominal examination

2.62 Poor fetal growth can be confirmed by:
- **A** serial human placental lactogen levels
- **B** presence of oligohydramnios
- **C** serial plasma oestriol estimations
- **D** diagnosis of pre-eclampsia
- **E** abnormal lecithin-sphingomyelin ratio

2.63 Annette is likely to be:
- **A** advised to rest at home
- **B** provided with a low sodium diet
- **C** asked to keep a fetal activity chart
- **D** given a daily cardiotocograph
- **E** admitted to a consultant obstetric unit

2.64 Intrauterine growth retardation may be associated with:
- **A** persistent hypertension
- **B** severe placental abruption
- **C** placental infarction
- **D** placental dysfunction
- **E** poorly controlled diabetes mellitus

(*answers overleaf*)

2.61 **A D**

An ultrasound scan in early pregnancy provides an accurate baseline with which to compare later clinical and ultrasonic examinations. In late pregnancy ultrasound examination remains the most effective way to estimate the duration of pregnancy.

2.62 **A C**

Oligohydramnios may indicate fetal abnormality such as renal agenesis or severe polycystic kidneys.
The liquor lecithin-sphingomyelin ratio is an indicator of fetal lung maturity, and may be important if poor fetal growth leads to the necessity to deliver the baby prematurely.

2.63 **C D E**

Fetal activity as detected by the mother herself and cardiotocography is an effective and non-invasive method of monitoring fetal well-being. As she has an active toddler, it is unlikely that resting at home will be very effective.

2.64 **A B C D E**

Intrauterine growth retardation may result from *all* these conditions, although poorly controlled diabetes is commonly associated with large, overweight babies.

SECTION III
TRUE OR FALSE? Questions 2.65–2.77

Indicate whether you think the statements listed below are true or false.

2.65 **Twin pregnancy occurs approximately 1:80 pregnancies.**

2.66 **Uniovular twins are 3–4 times as common as binovular twins.**

2.67 **Polyhydramnios is present in approximately 10–20 per cent of twin pregnancies.**

2.68 **In 80 per cent of twins, both are vertex presentations.**

2.69 **Intrapartum hypoxia is usually more severe with the first twin.**

2.70 **A missed abortion is termed a carneous mole if it is retained in the uterus for several weeks or more.**

2.71 **Glycosuria in pregnancy is associated with hyperemesis gravidarum.**

2.72 **The fetal head usually engages by 37 weeks in the primigravida.**

2.73 **Pregnancy is considered to be prolonged if labour has not commenced by 42 weeks.**

2.74 **A bacterial count of more than 100 000 organisms per ml is diagnostic of asymptomatic bacteriuria.**

2.75 **Serial urinary or plasma oestriol estimations reflect placental function.**

2.76 **All patients should attend the prenatal clinic weekly between 36 weeks and term.**

2.77 **Breast tenderness and enlargement may be one of the earliest signs of pregnancy.**

(*answers overleaf*)

2.65 **True**

2.66 **False**
Binovular twins account for 70–75 per cent of all twins.

2.67 **True**

2.68 **False**
Both twins present by the vertex in only 40–45 per cent of cases. Therefore almost 60 per cent of twins have one or more malpresentation.

2.69 **False**
Intrapartum hypoxia is generally more severe with the *second* twin.

2.70 **True**
A carneous mole results from a missed abortion retained in utero, where repeated haemorrhages into the chorio-decidual space eventually surround the blighted ovum, giving it a characteristic fleshy appearance. The treatment is to evacuate the uterus either surgically or by using oxytocic drugs.

2.71 **False**
Glycosuria is probably commoner in the pregnant than the non-pregnant state, due to marked increase in the glomerular filtration rate, or due to established or gestational diabetes mellitus

2.72 **True**

2.73 **True**
Provided that the original expected date of delivery was accurate.

2.74 **True**

2.75 **True**
In actual fact they reflect the function of the feto-placental unit.

2.76 **True**

2.77 **True**

SECTION IV
MATCHING ITEMS Questions 2.78–2.86

Match the items in Group 1 with the most appropriate item in Group 2. (Each item in Group 2 may only be used once.)

2.78 Match the items in Group 1 with the most appropriate condition in Group 2.

Group 1		*Group 2*
(i) low fat diet	**A**	iron deficiency anaemia
(ii) hydrops fetalis	**B**	rhesus iso-immunisation
(iii) clomiphene ('Clomid')	**C**	thalassaemia minor
(iv) ferrous gluconate	**D**	sub-fertility
	E	heartburn

2.79 Match the anaemias in Group 1 with the most appropriate item in Group 2.

Group 1		*Group 2*
(i) hypochromic, microcytic	**A**	negroid races
(ii) macrocytic, megaloblastic anaemia	**B**	sarcoidosis
	C	iron deficiency
(iii) sickle cell anaemia	**D**	folic acid deficiency
(iv) thalassaemia minor	**E**	mediterranean races

2.80 Match the items in Group 1 with the most appropriate item in Group 2.

Group 1		*Group 2*
(i) morning sickness	**A**	four weeks of pregnancy
(ii) uterus palpable abdominally	**B**	six weeks of pregnancy
(iii) amenorrhoea	**C**	12 weeks of pregnancy
(iv) 'quickening'	**D**	16–18 weeks of pregnancy
	E	20–24 weeks of pregnancy

2.81 Match the items in Group 1 with the most appropriate item in Group 2.

Group 1		*Group 2*
(i) pre-diabetes	**A**	increased glomerular filtration rate
(ii) glycosuria		
(iii) oligohydramnios	**B**	unstable lie
(iv) polyhydramnios	**C**	amenorrhoea
	D	large babies (> 4 kg)
	E	renal agenesis

(*answers overleaf*)

2.78
(i) **E**
(ii) **B**
(iii) **D**
(iv) **A**

2.79
(i) **C**
(ii) **D**
(iii) **A**
(iv) **E**

2.80
(i) **B**
(ii) **C**
(iii) **A**
(iv) **D**

2.81
(i) **D**
(ii) **A**
(iii) **E**
(iv) **B**

2.82 Match the drugs in Group 1 with the condition they are commonly used to treat in Group 2.

Group 1	*Group 2*
(i) nystatin	**A** heartburn
(ii) methyldopa (Aldomet)	**B** premature labour
(iii) antacids	**C** gonorrhoea
(iv) ritodrine (Yutopar)	**D** candidiasis
	E essential hypertension

2.83 Match the items in Group 1 with the most appropriate item in Group 2

Group 1	*Group 2*
(i) untreated diabetes	**A** rheumatic fever
(ii) proteinuria	**B** retention of urine
(iii) retroverted gravid uterus	**C** chronic nephritis
(iv) mitral stenosis	**D** infertility
	E achlorhydria

2.84 Match the items in Group 1 with the most suitable item in Group 2.

Group 1	*Group 2*
(i) frequency of micturition at 12 weeks	**A** oestrogen production
	B hypotension
(ii) fall in haemoglobin level	**C** uterine enlargement
(iii) growth of breast tissue	**D** increased blood volume
(iv) inferior vena caval compression	**E** chorionic gonadotrophin

2.85 Match the items in Group 1 with the most suitable item in Group 2.

Group 1	*Group 2*
(i) hydatidiform mole	**A** placental function test
(ii) human placental lactogen	**B** multiple pregnancy
(iii) chorion carcinoma	**C** metronidazole
(iv) folic acid deficiency	**D** increased urinary levels of chorionic gonadotrophin
	E methotrexate

2.86 Match the items in Group 1 with the most suitable item in Group 2.

Group 1	*Group 2*
(i) heartburn	**A** Shirodkar suture
(ii) fluid 'thrill'	**B** gastric reflux
(iii) cervical incompetence	**C** elevated blood pressure
(iv) pre-eclampsia	**D** polyhydramnios
	E vulval varicosities

(*answers overleaf*)

2.82
(i) **D**
(ii) **E**
(iii) **A**
(iv) **B**

2.83
(i) **D**
(ii) **C**
(iii) **B**
(iv) **A**

2.84
(i) **C**
(ii) **D**
(iii) **A**
(iv) **B**

2.85
(i) **D**
(ii) **A**
(iii) **E**
(iv) **B**

Hydatidiform mole is a potentially pre-malignant growth, which gives a positive pregnancy test even when the urine has been greatly diluted. This is due to the vast amounts of chorionic gonadotrophin produced by the mole. A chorion carcinoma is a folic acid dependent neoplasm, which although highly malignant, responds well to treatment with methotrexate, as this is a folic acid antagonist.

2.86
(i) **B**
(ii) **D**
(iii) **A**
(iv) **C**

SECTION V
ASSERTION/REASON/Questions 2.87–2.92

A Assertion true, reason is a true statement, and reason is the *correct* reason.
B Assertion and reason are both true, but reason is *not* the correct reason.
C Assertion is true, but reason is a false statement.
D Assertion is false, but reason true.
E Both are false.

Using the above criteria answer the following questions:

2.87 **Varicose veins of legs and vulva occur more commonly during pregnancy**
because
there is increased muscle tone due to circulating oxytocin.

2.88 **Placental localisation by ultrasound should never be done prior to amniocentesis**
because
rhesus iso-immunisation can occur if the placenta is punctured during the amniocentesis.

2.89 **Placental abruption is associated with a high perinatal loss**
because
the placenta is situated in the upper uterine segment.

2.90 **It is advisable to treat patients suffering from thalassaemia minor, with high doses of iron**
because
they can only utilise small amounts of iron, and the remainder may be laid down in the tissues and become toxic.

2.91 **A very careful menstrual history should be taken at the booking clinic**
because
it will help to establish an accurate expected date of delivery.

2.92 **Oligohydramnios may occur with a large meningomyelocele**
because
the fetus with an open neural tube defect does not secrete urine.

(*answers overleaf*)

2.87 **C**
Smooth muscle fibres such as those in the vein walls are *relaxed* during pregnancy, probably due to the large increase in circulating steroids.

2.88 **D**
Placental localisation by ultrasound should *always* take place prior to amniocentesis, so that placental damage may be avoided.

2.89 **B**
In placental abruption, the placenta *is* normally situated, but the increased perinatal loss, is due to placental separation and vasospasm which leads to severe fetal hypoxia and its sequelae.

2.90 **D**
Thalassaemic patients must *not* be given large doses of iron. If their anaemia in pregnancy becomes severe, then a blood transfusion may be given.

2.91 **A**

2.92 **E**
An *excess* of liquor amnii (polyhydramnios) may occur with open neural tube defects such as meningomyelocele or anencephaly, because persistent leakage of cerebrospinal fluid into the liquor alters the balance of the liquor volume. The fetal kidneys usually secrete urine normally, and this is passed into the liquor, forming a significant proportion of the liquor volume in the second half of pregnancy.

SECTION VI
COMPLETION ITEMS Questions 2.93–2.104

Supply the missing word (s) in the following statements:

2.93 **Pigmentation of facial skin in pregnancy is known as_______ and this pigmentation, probably due to increased steroid activity, can also be seen in the_____________________ on the abdomen, and_____________________of the breast.**

2.94 **In eclampsia, a_____________________catheter is usually inserted into the urinary bladder, so that the____________ can be monitored, and the degree of proteinuria assessed.**

2.95 **When an ectopic pregnancy occurs, the fertilised ovum may embed in the_____________________, the ____________ or the_____________________.**

2.96 **Bleeding from a cervical polyp may be termed____________ antepartum haemorrhage.**

2.97 **The commonest cause of a high head at term is an____.**

2.98 **Negro women should always be tested for______________ in early pregnancy.**

2.99 **Where a vaginal delivery is anticipated with a breech presentation,_____________________should be performed prior to labour.**

2.100 **Occult oedema may be diagnosed by detecting excessive____.**

2.101 **If a woman has a regular menstrual cycle lasting 42 days, (instead of the normal 28 days), it will be the____________ half of the cycle which will be extended by two weeks.**

2.102 **Total weight gain in pregnancy should not exceed___________ and in the last half of pregnancy, weekly weight gain should not exceed____.**

(answers overleaf)

2.93 a Chloasma (or the 'mask of pregnancy')
b Linea nigra
c Primary and secondary areolae

2.94 a Self-retaining
b Urinary output

2.95 a Fallopian (uterine) tube
b Ovary
c Abdominal cavity

2.96 Incidental

2.97 Occipito-posterior position

2.98 Sickle cell anaemia

2.99 Erect lateral X-ray pelvimetry

2.100 Weight gain

2.101 First (Proliferative phase)

2.102 a 11–13 kg
b 500 g

2.103 To calculate the expected date of delivery by Naegele's formula, take Day__________________of the patient's last normal period, and add__________________days plus__________________months.

2.104 Polyhydramnios occurs with__________________ because the fetus does not swallow the liquor amnii.

(answers overleaf)

2.103 a One
b Seven
c Nine

2.104 Oesophageal atresia
The liquor volume is finely balanced and easily upset. If the fetus cannot swallow liquor, then liquor will not be absorbed through the fetal gastro-intestinal tract, and so an excess of liquor may result, as input will exceed output.
Babies born to mothers with significant polyhydramnios should have a large gauge oesophageal tube passed at delivery to exclude oesophageal atresia.

CASE HISTORY

At her routine antenatal clinic visit, Karen, a grande multipara, is found to be clinically large for her dates. As she booked late she did not have an early ultrasound scan.

Supply the missing word(s) in the following statements:

2.105 When questioned, Karen agreed that her last menstrual period had been more scanty than usual. This could indicate that instead of being normal menstrual bleeding, Karen's loss could have been due to__________ or__________bleeding.

2.106 In order to estimate her gestation as accurately as possible, Karen then had an__________. This can also detect open neural tube defects such as__________. On adominal examination these may well be associated with an excess of__________.

2.107 Some soft tissue defects such as__________ and__________can also be associated with polyhydramnios, but these are not so easy to diagnose.

2.108 The other major cause of the 'large-for-dates' uterus is__________, the commonest form of which is__________pregnancy which has an incidence of approximately 1:80.

(*answers overleaf*)

2.105 a Decidual (bleeding)
b Implantation (bleeding)

2.106 a Ultrasound scan
b Anencephaly, meningomyelocele
c Liquor amnii

2.107 a Exomphalos (a protrusion of intestines through an opening in the abdominal wall at the umbilicus), or gastroschisis (a major abdominal wall defect with protrusion of intestines and other abdominal organs)
b oesophageal atresia

2.108 a Multiple pregnancy
b Twin

PREGNANCY

The following questions are taken from recent examination papers set by the English National Board.

1. Essay questions

**Discuss the value of parentcraft.
How may a midwife arrange a series of parentcraft classes?
What subjects should be included in these sessions? (1983)**

Describe in detail how a midwife would carry out a routine antenatal examination of a woman expecting her first baby, when the period of gestation is 38 weeks. What advice might be particularly appropriate at this stage of her pregnancy? (1983)

**Anaemia is a common complication of pregnancy.
Outline the possible explanation for this. In what way can anaemia be prevented? What may be the effects of untreated iron deficiency anaemia in pregnancy? (1983)**

What is pre-eclampsia? How can a midwife assist in the recognition and management of such a case? (1983)

Describe the anxieties a young married woman may have when pregnant for the first time. What advice and help can the midwife give to this woman? (1983)

Discuss the social, medical and obstetric effects of sexually transmitted diseases in the pregnant woman. (1983)

What would make you suspect a multiple pregnancy? Discuss the antenatal complications and management of such a pregnancy. (1983)

Discuss the reasons for obtaining information from a woman in early pregnancy regarding her medical, social, emotional and obstetric background. (1983)

Mrs Gilbert is now 34 weeks pregnant. This is her third pregnancy and she has two children aged 2 years and 6 years. She calls you to her home because she is bleeding per vaginam. Discuss your immediate management. Outline the subsequent care and the possible outcomes of this pregnancy. (1983)

A woman who has had a previous stillbirth attends the antenatal clinic for the first time early in her second pregnancy. What is the importance of the first visit for this woman? (1983)

Discuss the role of the midwife in identifying 'high risk' women during the antenatal period. (1984)

Why do some women fail to receive adequate antenatal care? What can the midwife do to improve the 'take-up' and quality of antenatal care? (1984)

Women may develop vaginal discharges in pregnancy. How does the midwife identify the different types?
How would they be managed and what complications may occur? (1984)

What is the role of the midwife in providing antenatal care for a pregnant woman?
How may other members of the health team be involved? (1984)

Identify the causes of bleeding from the genital tract before the 28th week of pregnancy.
Describe the management, care and support of a woman threatening to abort at 24 week's gestation. (1984)

Define grande multiparity.
What potential problems place these women at risk?
Describe the management of these problems during pregnancy. (1984)

Pregnancy is a period of change, physical, psychological and emotional. How can a midwife assist a woman to adapt to these changes? (1984)
'Midwives should participate in all aspects of prenatal care'. (The Role of the Midwife, 1983)
Explain how the midwife should be involved in this care. (1984)

Discuss the management and care of a woman whose uterine size is smaller than expected for the estimated gestational age. (1984)

Discuss the significance of blood tests carried out in pregnancy. (1985)

List the conditions which may cause hypertension in pregnancy.
Describe the midwife's role in the recognition of pre-eclampsia.
How may pre-eclampsia affect the outcome for both mother and baby? (1985)

2. Write briefly on each of the following subjects:
The value of 'shared' antenatal care (1983)
Minor disorders of pregnancy (1983)
Causes of hypertension in pregnancy (1983)
Weight gain during pregnancy (1983)
Causes of vaginal discharge in pregnancy (1983)
Antenatal clinic defaulters (1983)
Recognition of polyhydramnios (1983)
Causes of vomiting in pregnancy (1983)

Diagnosis of multiple pregnancy (1983)
Signs and symptons of impending eclampsia (1983)
Ectopic pregnancy (1983)
Use of ultrasound in pregnancy (1983)
Herpes infections in pregnancy (1983)
Obesity in pregnancy (1983)
Indications for amniocentesis in the first half of pregnancy (1983)
Effects of pregnancy on a woman with diabetes mellitus (1983)
Methods of assessment of gestation (1983)
Proteinuria during pregnancy (1983)
The value of continuity of care during the antenatal period (1984)
Diagnosis of placental abruption (1984)
The consumption of alcohol during pregnancy (1984)
Pre-conception care (1984)
Diagnosis of pregnancy (1984)
Unstable lie (1984)
Sickle cell anaemia (1984)
The value of midwives' clinics (1984)
Estimation of expected date of delivery (1984)
Constipation during pregnancy (1984)
Ketonuria during pregnancy (1984)
Sexual intercourse during pregnancy (1984)
Megaloblastic anaemia (1984)
Drug abuse during pregnancy (1984)
Diagnosis of intra-uterine death (1984)
Importance of recording blood pressure during pregnancy (1984)
Problems associated with a retroverted uterus in pregnancy (1985)
Recognition of eclampsia (1985)
The 'Warnock Report' (1985)
Transverse lie (1985)
Acquired Immune Deficiency Syndrome (AIDS) (1985)
The law in relation to termination of pregnancy (1985)
Pica (1985)
Polyhydramnios (1985)

3. Labour

SECTION I
SINGLE RESPONSE MULTIPLE CHOICE QUESTIONS Questions 3.1–3.13

Select a *single* correct response to each of the following questions.

3.1 The duration of labour is calculated from the time when:
- **A** the membranes rupture
- **B** a 'show' is passed
- **C** backache is first noticed
- **D** regular contractions begin

3.2 The most certain sign of the onset of labour is:
- **A** a 'show'
- **B** regular contractions
- **C** dilatation of the cervical os
- **D** rupture of the membranes

3.3 The onset of the second stage of labour can be positively confirmed when:
- **A** the mother feels expulsive contractions
- **B** the mother vomits
- **C** no cervix is felt on vaginal examination
- **D** the fetal head is visible in the vagina

3.4 Immediately after delivery of the placenta and membranes, the midwife's first priority must be to:
- **A** give the baby to its mother to hold
- **B** inspect the perineum for lacerations
- **C** examine the placenta
- **D** check that the uterus is well contracted

(*answers overleaf*)

3.1 **D**

3.2 **C**

Significant cervical dilatation definitely confirms the onset of labour.

3.3 **C**

The mother may feel an overwhelming desire to bear down late in the first stage of labour, and the presenting part can sometimes be seen in the vagina prior to full dilatation of the cervix, e.g. when a 'lip' of cervix persists.

3.4 **D**

All the other options are important, and must be undertaken as speedily as possible by the midwife. However, her first priority is to prevent haemorrhage by ensuring that the uterus remains well contracted.

3.5 Pethidine is preferred to morphine in labour because it:
A does not affect the bowel
B causes less respiratory depression in the fetus
C acts more quickly
D is a more powerful analgesic

3.6 Women in labour may be given an antacid to prevent:
A heartburn
B nausea and vomiting
C gastric reflux
D Mendelson's syndrome

3.7 Ketonuria in labour is the result of one of the following being metabolised:
A carbohydrates
B fats
C proteins
D amino acids

3.8 The normal range for the fetal heart rate in beats per minute is:
A 120–160
B 130–150
C 100–160
D 120–180

3.9 A newly delivered woman (in a consultant unit) starts to bleed torrentially before the delivery of the placenta. The midwife is alone with her patient. Indicate in what order you would undertake the following action:
1 send for a doctor
2 rub up a contraction
3 give i.v. ergometrine
4 catheterise the bladder
A 1, 2, 4, 3
B 1, 4, 3, 2
C 2, 1, 3, 4
D 4, 3, 2, 1

3.10 If profuse bleeding *per vaginam* occurs during the third stage of labour in the presence of a well-contracted uterus, the cause is likely to be:
A uterine atony
B cervical lacerations
C placental site bleeding
D cervical polyp

(*answers overleaf*)

3.5 **B**

However, pethidine can depress the fetal respiratory centre, which may be severe enough to require the administration of a pure narcotic antagonist such as naloxone (Narcan Neonatal)

3.6 **D**

Many labouring women still receive an antacid preparation in labour to keep the stomach contents alkali and prevent the acid aspiration (Mendelson's) syndrome. However, some authorities think that regular antacid therapy can lead to reflux hyperacidity, and only give antacids prior to general anaesthesia. An alternative preventive measure is to reduce the production of gastric acid by using a drug such as ranitidine ('Zantac')

3.7 **B**

3.8 **A**

3.9 **C**

3.10 **B**

Or a severe posterior vaginal wall laceration, which may extend up into the fornices and involve large vessels.

3.11 In a face presentation, the denominator is the:
A bregma
B glabella
C sinciput
D mentum

3.12 Patients receiving i.v. syntocinon in labour must be carefully watched for:
A a fall in blood pressure
B prolapse of the umbilical cord
C tonic uterine contractions
D maternal exhaustion

3.13 A constriction ring is:
A incoordinate uterine action
B retraction ring
C localised tonic spasm of uterine muscle
D Bandl's ring

(answers overleaf)

3.11 **D**

Mentum is the Latin for the chin.

3.12 **C**

Intravenous syntocinon can easily overstimulate the uterine muscle, and hypertonic contractions can cause fetal distress, as the oxygen supply to the fetus is so diminished, or in extreme cases a ruptured uterus and/or fetal death.

3.13 **C**

Constriction ring can occur with the fetus inside the uterus, or after delivery, when it may be the cause of a retained placenta. (*N.B.* Retraction ring is the normal, physiological demarcation between the upper and lower uterine segments. It is most marked at the end of the first stage of labour when the upper segment is thickened, and the lower segment well thinned out. In obstructed labour, this retraction ring may become even more pronounced as the lower segment becomes pathologically thin prior to an impending rupture of the uterus, and it is then known as Bandl's ring.)

SECTION II
MULTIPLE RESPONSE QUESTIONS Questions 3.14–3.44

Select any number of correct responses between 1–5.

3.14 In normal labour:
A there is steady cervical dilatation and descent of the presenting part
B the fetal heart rate may vary between 100–160 beats per minute
C the liquor may be meconium stained
D uterine contractions increase in strength, duration and frequency
E the blood pressure may fall significantly

3.15 The second stage of labour:
A must always be confirmed by vaginal examination
B should not last longer than one hour
C may be heralded by expulsive contractions, and a gaping anus
D must be confirmed vaginally in breech presentation
E is confirmed when the presenting part is visible

3.16 The third stage:
A lasts from the birth of the baby until six hours after delivery
B if conducted, (without any intervention), by maternal effort, lasts approximately 20–40 minutes
C with active management, is completed in 5–10 minutes
D involves the separation and expulsion of the placenta, and the control of haemorrhage
E is the most dangerous stage of labour for the mother

3.17 The Midwives Rules of the UK Central Council for Nursing Midwifery and Health Visiting allow a midwife to:
A administer ergometrine intravenously in emergency
B suture the perineum
C induce epidural analgesia
D 'top-up' epidural analgesia
E intubate a severely asphyxiated neonate

3.18 Oxytocin:
A is called Syntocinon in its synthetic form
B acts on smooth muscle, particularly the uterus
C midwives may prescribe Syntocinon for induction of labour
D acts principally on the central nervous system
E five units is given in combination with ergometrine 0.5 mg as Syntometrine

(*answers overleaf*)

3.14 **A D**

The normal fetal heart range is 120–160 b.p.m., and the liquor is not meconium stained unless the fetus has suffered a hypoxic episode. The blood pressure should not fall signficantly unless the mother has an epidural block, caval compression (supine hypotension) from lying flat on her back, or is shocked for some other reason.

3.15 **B C D**

The second stage is frequently diagnosed by vaginal examination, but it is not always necessary, except where there is a breech presentation. In the latter, it is vital that the mother should not be allowed to use her expulsive contractions until full dilatation of the cervix is definitely confirmed. Remember that it is possible to see the presenting part (often a large caput) and still not have complete cervical dilatation, e.g. there may be an oedematous anterior lip of cervix. It is generally unwise for the second stage of labour to be prolonged, as sustained uterine contractions reduce the oxygen supply to the fetus. In the presence of effective, expulsive contractions, the presenting part should advance steadily, and delivery can usually be achieved within an hour.

3.16 **B C D E**

The third stage of labour lasts from the birth of the infant until the placenta and membranes are expelled. If managed physiologically, *without* the use of oxytocics and controlled cord traction, it will take approximately 20–40 minutes.

3.17 **A B D E**

If she has been properly instructed, the midwife may 'top-up' epidural blocks and, in an emergency, administer i.v. ergometrine or intubate a severely asphyxiated baby. She may also suture the perineum, if she has been properly instructed, and if the obstetrician is prepared to take responsibility for her undertaking this procedure.

3.18 **A B E**

Only doctors may prescribe the use of Syntocinon for the induction or acceleration of labour.

3.19 Pethidine:

A has an anti-emetic effect
B may be prescribed in labour by a community midwife
C acts as an analgesic and antispasmodic
D can depress the fetal respiratory centre
E raises the blood pressure

3.20 Primary postpartum haemorrhage:

A is less severe where there is a maternal anaemia
B is usually a loss of more than 500 ml of blood from the genital tract
C can be caused by cervical lacerations
D is commonly associated with uterine atony
E occurs during the 6 hours immediately following delivery of the baby

3.21 Damage to the perineal body is more common with:

A a well-flexed head
B rigid perineum
C face to pubes delivery
D previous episiotomy
E grande multiparity

3.22 A generous medio-lateral episiotomy will cut fibres of the following muscles:

A pubococcygeus
B bulbocavernosus
C ischiocavernosus
D external anal sphincter
E transverse perineal muscles

3.23 The Midwives Rules (UK Central Council) allow a midwife to administer a local anaesthetic to the perineal area, prior to episiotomy. This may be:

A 5 ml lignocaine 1 per cent
B 10 ml lignocaine 0.5 per cent
C 10 ml lignocaine 1 per cent
D 5 ml Marcain (bupivacaine) 0.5 per cent
E 10 ml Marcain (bupivacaine) 0.25 per cent

3.24 A third degree tear:

A involves severe damage to the anal sphincter
B may extend into the lower bowel
C can lead to a vesico-vaginal fistula
D may be repaired by a midwife
E if badly repaired can cause incontinence of faeces

(*answers overleaf*)

3.19 **B C D**
Pethidine does not raise the blood pressure, but has a tendency to make some women vomit, which is why it is frequently administered with an anti-emetic drug such as promazine hydrochloride ('Sparine')

3.20 **B C D**
Postpartum haemorrhage is bleeding from the genital tract, usually in excess of 500 ml, but may be a lesser amount if it causes the patient's condition to deteriorate, e.g. with a severe maternal anaemia.
Primary postpartum haemorrhage occurs during the first 24 hours following delivery, and secondary postpartum haemorrhage between 24 hours and 6 weeks.

3.21 **B C D**
A generous episiotomy will be needed for both a rigid perineum and many face-to-pubes deliveries. In the former this is because there can be delay which could lead to fetal hypoxia, and the perineum may then rupture at delivery. In the latter, it is because the wider diameters of the deflexed fetal head distend the soft tissues at the introitus and can cause severe lacerations. Good judgment will be needed where there has been previous scarring, but in some cases an episiotomy will be necessary to prevent a major laceration, as fibrous scar tissue is inelastic.

3.22 **A B E**

3.23 **A B**

3.24 **A B E**
A third degree tear must be expertly repaired by *an experienced* doctor. An inadequate repair may lead to a recto-vaginal fistula and faecal incontinence.

3.25 The Midwives Rules (UK Central Council), together with the controlled drugs legislation and the Medicines Act 1968, permit community midwives to prescribe the following drugs in the course of their professional practice:

A pethidine hydrochloride
B pentazocine (Fortral)
C Syntometrine
D promazine (Sparine)
E naloxone (Narcan)

3.26 The following inhalational analgesia machines are approved by the UK Central Council for use by midwives:

A Tecota Mark 6
B Cardiff inhaler
C Emotril
D Entonox
E Lucy Baldwin

(*answers overleaf*)

3.25 **A B C D E**

Remember that only midwives working as independent practitioners in the community have limited prescribing rights for drugs. In hospital *all* drugs are legally prescribed by the doctor. Pethidine is the only *Controlled* drug which may be prescribed by a midwife, and its use is governed by the Misuse of Drugs Regulations (1973–74).

3.26 **B D**

The Tecota Mark 6 and Emotril machines dispensing trichloroethylene (Trilene) are no longer approved for use, and 'Trilene' has been withdrawn from the list of approved inhalational analgesic agents for use by midwives. The Cardiff inhaler dispenses methoxyflurane (Penthrane) 0.35 per cent in air, and the Entonox apparatus is used for nitrous oxide with oxygen (50 per cent/ 50 per cent). The Lucy Baldwin apparatus is not approved for unsupervised use by midwives, as it dispenses nitrous oxide and oxygen in variable amounts—up to 70 per cent nitrous oxide with only 30 per cent oxygen.

CASE HISTORY

Following a normal delivery, and routine administration of i.m. Syntometrine 1 ml with the birth of the anterior shoulder, the midwife in an isolated general practitioner unit, fails to deliver the placenta. After 15 minutes, there is brisk bleeding *per vaginam*.

The following three questions relate to the above information.

3.27 Which of the following may be the cause of the retained placenta?

A Bandl's ring
B full bladder
C partial placenta accreta
D multiple pregnancy
E constriction ring

3.28 What *immediate* action should the midwife take?

A give an oxytocic drug
B send for the general practitioner
C catheterise the bladder
D give rectal tap water
E send for the obstetric 'flying squad'

3.29 The mother has already lost approximately 2 litres of blood when the obstetrician arrives. His *immediate* action will be to:

A set up an i.v. dextrose/saline infusion
B give a blood transfusion
C take blood for cross-matching
D transfer the mother to hospital *at once*
E carry out manual removal of placenta

3.30 Shoulder presentation produces an ill-fitting presenting part, with the following possible complications:

A vasa praevia
B cord prolapse
C footling breech
D early rupture of the membranes
E arm prolapse

(*answers overleaf*)

3.27 **B C E**
For information on Bandl's ring, see p. 102.

3.28 **A C E**
If possible, inform the general practitioner also, but send for the obstetric 'flying squad' first!

3.29 **B C E**
As an i.v. line is set up, blood can be taken for ABO group and cross-matching, and then whenever possible blood should be transfused. Most obstetric 'flying squads' carry two units of Group O rhesus negative (universal donor) blood, but if blood is not available then plasma or one of the plasma expanders should be used. Whenever possible the placenta should be removed *before* transfer to hospital, as torrential haemorrhage can occur in transit. The Confidential Enquiry into Maternal Deaths has shown that fatalities occur when moribund women are subjected to an ambulance ride before proper resuscitative treatment has been instituted.

3.30 **B D E**
Any ill-fitting presenting part incurs an increased risk of early rupture of the membranes and a possible cord prolapse, but the gravest complication of a shoulder presentation is a prolapsed arm.

3.31 Excessive traction during a difficult forceps delivery can result in the following birth injuries:
A depressed fracture of the skull
B Erb's palsy
C talipes equinovarus
D facial palsy
E syndactyly

3.32 Placenta accreta:
A is associated with postpartum haemorrhage
B causes hydatidiform mole
C may lead to retained placenta
D will necessitate manual removal
E is a morbidly adherent placenta

3.33 Acute inversion of the uterus is usually associated with:
A antepartum haemorrhage
B folate deficiency
C lax uterine muscles
D uncontrolled cord traction
E grande multiparity

3.34 In acute inversion, the uterus should be replaced:
A immediately, by hand
B after 24 hours
C following laparotomy
D by Credé's manoeuvre
E by hydrostatic pressure

3.35 Incoordinate uterine action may be characterised by:
A prolonged labour
B polarity
C severe backache
D slow cervical dilatation
E increased incidence of fetal distress

3.36 Occipito-posterior positions may be diagnosed on abdominal examination by finding:
A the fetal heart loudest above the umbilicus
B a slight saucer-like depression below the umbilicus
C a large number of fetal parts anteriorly
D the sinciput and occiput at the same level
E a well flexed head

(*answers overleaf*)

3.31 **A B D**

Badly applied forceps can produce skull fractures, and strong traction may damage the 7th cranial (facial) nerve, (to produce a Bell's palsy), or the brachial plexus, which may cause an Erb's or a Klumpke's palsy, depending on which nerve roots are affected. Except in a few cases, these palsies resolve spontaneously.

3.32 **A C D E**

A completely adherent placenta accreta will not bleed, but this is rare, because the majority are only partially adherent, and then the area of normal placenta separates, causing the exposed maternal vessels in the placental bed to bleed profusely. Provided that the chorionic villi have only penetrated the basal layer of the decidua or superficial myometrium, manual removal of placenta will usually be possible. In rare cases, deep penetration of the myometrium can occur (placenta increta or percreta) and in these cases hysterectomy may be necessary.

3.33 **C D E**

When active management of the third stage is practised, acute inversion of the uterus is generally due to a mismanaged third stage with *uncontrolled* cord traction, and a poorly contracted uterus. Occasionally, it may be spontaneous—usually in a grande multipara with lax abdominal and pelvic floor muscles.

3.34 **A E**

It is important that the doctor or midwife attempts *immediate* replacement of the uterus before tonic spasm of the lower segment intervenes. Any delay will lead to the need for a general anaesthetic, and possibly the use of hydrostatic pressure. The patient will be profoundly shocked, and can even die.

3.35 **A C D E**

Classically, incoordinate uterine action produces strong, painful (but not polarised) contractions, which fail to dilate the cervix efficiently.
This leads to a long, painful labour, often complicated by maternal and fetal distress. However, epidural analgesia relieves the pain, and improves the efficiency of the contractions, thus preventing a long labour in many cases.

3.36 **B C D**

As the head is usually deflexed (military attitude) in occipito-posterior positions, and seldom engaged before labour is established, it may be possible to recognise that the occiput and sinciput are both on the same level.

3.37 When hypotonic uterine action occurs, there is often:
- **A** precipitate delivery
- **B** prolonged labour
- **C** i.v. Syntocinon
- **D** severe backache
- **E** tonic contractions

3.38 The following manoeuvres may be undertaken by a midwife during an emergency breech delivery:
- **A** Løvset's manoeuvre
- **B** jaw flexion/shoulder traction
- **C** Burns-Marshall manoeuvre
- **D** internal podalic version
- **E** Paget's manoeuve

3.39 Face presentation
- **A** has an engaging diameter of 9.5 cm (approx.)
- **B** almost always delivers vaginally
- **C** may ensue following an occipito-posterior position
- **D** frequently occurs with anencephaly
- **E** has the sinciput as the denominator

3.40 Brow presentation:
- **A** reduces the risk of cord prolapse
- **B** is usually delivered by caesarean section
- **C** has no true mechanism
- **D** is a favourable presentation
- **E** will not usually enter the pelvis because the engaging diameter is the mento-vertical (13.3 cm)

3.41 The main factors influencing the successful outcome of a 'trial of labour' are:
- **A** haemoglobin level
- **B** mobility of the pelvic joints
- **C** Osiander's sign
- **D** uterine action
- **E** moulding' of the fetal head

3.42 Cord prolapse is associated with:
- **A** flexed breech presentation
- **B** extended breech presentation
- **C** oligohydramnios
- **D** circumvallate placenta
- **E** unstable lie

(*answers overleaf*)

3.37 **B C**
Hypotonic uterine action usually produces a long, but not particularly painful labour. Intravenous Syntocinon is frequently used to improve the uterine action, and shorten the labour.

3.38 **A B C**
Jaw flexion/shoulder traction (Mauriceau-Smellie-Veit manoeuvre), and the Burns-Marshall manoeuvre, are both recognised procedures for delivering the aftercoming head of a breech. These, and Løvset's manoeuvre to deliver extended arms, may be used by a midwife undertaking an emergency breech delivery.

3.39 **A C D**
A face presentation has an engaging diameter (sub-mento-bregmatic) of 9.5 cm and the denominator is the chin (mentum). Anencephaly is usually a primary face presentation, as there is little except the face to present. A secondary face presentation may follow an occipito-posterior position, where descent in labour occurs with complete extension of the head.

3.40 **B C E**
Brow presentation has no true mechanism, as the engaging diameter is generally too large to enter the pelvis, and so most are delivered by caesarean section. The high head and poorly fitting presenting part predispose to early rupture of the membranes and cord prolapse.

3.41 **B D E**
Trial of labour is carried out where there is a *known* minor degree of cephalo-pelvic disproportion, but if the uterine action is efficient and moulding of the fetal head, plus some 'give' in the pelvic joints occurs, then a safe, vaginal delivery should result.

3.42 **A E**
An extended breech often enters the pelvic brim, and is less likely to be associated with cord prolapse. Unstable lie is often seen with polyhydramnios and grande multiparity, and is a common cause of cord prolapse.

3.43 Cephalo-pelvic disproportion:
A is usually treated with an oxytocic infusion in labour
B generally leads to caesarean section
C is associated with eclampsia
D may be assessed by Munro-Kerr's method
E may be due to hydrocephaly

3.44 At a home confinement, the midwife can monitor the progress of labour by:
A abdominal palpation
B fetal heart rate
C maternal pulse
D length and strength of uterine contractions
E vaginal examination

(*answers overleaf*)

3.43 **B D E**

Moderate to severe disproportion is generally managed by elective caesarean section, but minor degrees may achieve vaginal delivery following a 'trial of labour'. Occasionally an oxytocin infusion is used, but enormous care must be taken, as obstructed labour and uterine rupture could result if obstetric judgment has been poor. Munro-Kerr devised a bi-manual method of assessing the degree of disproportion.

3.44 **A D E**

Descent of the presenting part can be measured by abdominal palpation and vaginal examination, where the station of the head in relation to the ischial spines can be assessed. Cervical effacement and dilatation are also measured, and the experienced midwife can use the pattern of contractions to help her assess progress in labour.

SECTION III
TRUE OR FALSE? Questions 3.45–3.57

Indicate if you think the statements listed below are true or false.

3.45 **In labour, the pelvic floor directs the leading part of the fetus forward, to lie under the symphysis pubis.**

3.46 **Oxytocic drugs tend to elevate the blood pressure.**

3.47 **Induction of labour is usually indicated with severe placental abruption.**

3.48 **Active management of the third stage of labour has reduced the incidence of postpartum haemorrhage.**

3.49 **On vaginal examination the anterior fontanelle can be felt when the head is well flexed.**

3.50 **In labour, frank meconium may indicate a breech presentation.**

3.51 **A woman in established labour should be encouraged to pass urine two-hourly.**

3.52 **Ritodrine (Yutopar) and salbutamol (Ventolin) are preparations which assist ripening of the cervix prior to induction of labour.**

3.53 **Reduced fetal activity, or excessive fetal movement, can be diagnostic signs of fetal distress.**

3.54 **A pudendal block using local anaesthetic, will produce a satisfactory regional anaesthesia for forceps delivery.**

3.55 **Vacuum (Ventouse) extraction may be used to expedite delivery during the later part of the first stage of labour.**

3.56 **A fetal scalp electrode produces a better fetal heart tracing on the cardiotocograph, than does an external transducer.**

(*answers overleaf*)

3.45 **True**

3.46 **True**
This is why they must be used with great care in hypertensive patients. However, their effect can often by usefully counteracted by the *hypotensive* effect of epidural analgesia.

3.47 **True**
Severe placental abruption has a poor fetal prognosis, and therefore artificial rupture of the membranes and vaginal delivery will often be the treatment of choice.

3.48 **True**

3.49 **False**
The anterior fontanelle is usually only felt when the head is *poorly* flexed (deflexed).

3.50 **True**

3.51 **True**
It is important for the smooth progress of labour to keep the bladder empty, if necessary resorting to catheterisation.

3.52 **False**
Ritodrine and salbutamol are both drugs used in an attempt to prevent premature labour. Intravaginal prostaglandins may be used to ripen an unfavourable cervix prior to induction of labour.

3.53 **True**

3.54 **True**
The local anaesthetic is injected around the ischial spines where the pudendal nerve re-enters the pelvis prior to dividing up to supply the vagina and perineal area.

3.55 **True**
The advantage of the vacuum extractor (Ventouse), is that it can be used during the first stage of labour, and can hasten cervical dilatation, as well as expedite the actual delivery.

3.56 **True**
It is also pleasanter for the mother, who does not have the discomfort of a tight belt and bulky transducer on her abdomen.

3.57 The use of pethidine by community midwives is governed by the Medicines Act 1968.

(answers overleaf)

3.57 **False**

The limited prescribing rights of the community midwife with regard to pethidine are written into the Misuse of Drugs Act 1971, and the Misuse of Drugs Regulations passed in 1973–74. The use of pethidine by midwives has been approved by the statutory body since 1939.

SECTION IV
MATCHING ITEMS Questions 3.58–3.66

Match the items in Group 1 with the most appropriate item in Group 2. (Each item in Group 2 may only be used *once*.)

3.58 Match the items in Group 1 with the most appropriate item in Group 2.

Group 1
(i) marcain
(ii) Penthrane
(iii) nitrous oxide and oxygen
(iv) lignocaine

Group 2
A 0.25 per cent
B 0.5 per cent
C 0.35 per cent
D 50 per cent/50 per cent
E 2 per cent

3.59 Match the items in Group 1 with most appropriate item in Group 2.

Group 1
(i) retraction
(ii) operculum
(iii) military attitude
(iv) episiotomy

Group 2
A perineal infiltration
B deflexion of the fetal head
C myometrium
D polarity
E show

3.60 Match the items in Group 1 with the most appropriate item in Group 2.

Group 1
(i) vasa praevia
(ii) Spalding's sign
(iii) anencephaly
(iv) brow presentation

Group 2
A lower segment caesarean section
B velamentous insertion of cord
C intra-uterine death
D primary face presentation
E Mendelson's syndrome

3.61 Match the items in Group 1 with the most appropriate item in Group 2.

Group 1
(i) high head
(ii) trial of scar
(iii) transverse lie
(iv) hypotonic uterine action

Group 2
A intravenous Syntocinon
B grande multiparity
C velamentous insertion of cord
D contracted pelvis
E previous hysterotomy

(*answers overleaf*

3.58
(i) **A**
(ii) **C**
(iii) **D**
(iv) **B**

3.59
(i) **C**
(ii) **E**
(iii) **B**
(iv) **A**

3.60
(i) **B**
(ii) **C**
(iii) **D**
(iv) **A**

3.61
(i) **D**
(ii) **E**
(iii) **B**
(iv) **A**

3.62 Match the items in Group 1 with the most appropriate item in Group 2.

Group 1		*Group 2*
(i) Løvset manoeuvre	A	cervical effacement
(ii) sub-mento-bregmatic diameter	B	extended arms
(iii) jaw flexion/shoulder traction	C	hypotension
(iv) Bishop's score	D	deflexed head
	E	face presentation

3.63 Match the items in Group 1 with the most appropriate item in Group 2.

Group 1		*Group 2*
(i) Bandl's ring	A	bupivacaine (Marcain)
(ii) caval compression	B	obstructed labour
(iii) epidural block	C	constriction ring
(iv) Burns-Marshall manoeuvre	D	aftercoming head of a breech
	E	hypotension

3.64 Match the drugs in Group 1 with the most appropriate dosage in Group 2.

Group 1		*Group 2*
(i) pethidine	A	0.02–0.04 mg
(ii) promazine (Sparine)	B	1–2 mg
(iii) naloxone (Narcan Neonatal)	C	100–150 mg
(iv) vitamin K_1 (Konakion)	D	0.5–1.0 mg
	E	25–50 mg

3.65 Match the items in Group 1 with the most appropriate item in Group 2.

Group 1		*Group 2*
(i) fetal scalp electrode	A	fetal blood sampling
(ii) amniotomy hook	B	Cardiff pump
(iii) Cusco's speculum	C	cardiotocography
(iv) pH meter	D	induction of labour
	E	high vaginal swab

3.66 With reference to vaginal examination in labour, match the items in Group 1 with the most appropriate item in Group 2.

Group 1		*Group 2*
(i) well-flexed head	A	anterior fontanelle
(ii) deflexed head	B	orbital ridges
(iii) brow presentation	C	posterior fontanelle
(iv) face presentation	D	gum margins
	E	occiput

(*answers overleaf*)

3.62
(i) **B**
(ii) **E**
(iii) **D**
Jaw flexion/shoulder traction is used to flex the deflexed (slightly extended) after-coming head of a breech presentation at delivery.
(iv) **A**

3.63
(i) **B**
(ii) **E**
(iii) **A**
(iv) **D**

3.64
(i) **C**
(ii) **E**
(iii) **A**
The dosage of naloxone (Narcan Neonatal) is 0.01 mg/kg body weight
(iv) **D**

3.65
(i) **C**
(ii) **D**
(iii) **E**
(iv) **A**

3.66
(i) **C**
(ii) **A**
(iii) **B**
(iv) **D**

SECTION V
ASSERTION/REASON Questions 3.67–3.73

Read carefully the five possible answers listed below marked **A, B, C, D, and E**. Select which is appropriate for the assertions and reasons which follow:

A Assertion true; reason is a true statement, and is the correct reason.
B Assertion and reason both true, but reason is *not* the correct reason.
C Assertion is true, but reason is a false statement.
D Assertion is false, but the reason is a true statement.
E Assertion and reason are both false.

3.67 **Solid food should be given during labour**
because
it helps to prevent the onset of ketonuria.

3.68 **Postpartum haemorrhage is always a potential danger following a twin delivery**
because
there is always placental dysfunction in multiple pregnancy.

3.69 **Occipito-posterior positions of the fetal head can cause delay in labour**
because
presenting diameters of the fetal skull are larger in occipito-posterior positions.

3.70 **Fetal blood sampling may be performed where fetal distress has been diagnosed by abnormal fetal heart patterns on a cardiotocograph**
because
it will confirm fetal hypoxia by detecting a raised blood pH.

3.71 **Caesarean section is often performed for a brow presentation**
because
the mento-vertical diameter of the fetal skull is too large to enter an average sized pelvis.

3.72 **A trial of labour should always be carried out in a consultant unit**
because
there is a known minor degree of cephalo-pelvic disproportion which may require expert obstetric intervention.

(*answers overleaf*)

3.67 **E**

Solids are rarely given to patients in labour nowadays because of the risks from a full stomach if unexpected general anaesthesia is required. Also the gastric motility and absorption of food from the stomach is greatly reduced, and feeding solid food to patients in labour will not necessarily prevent keto-acidosis.

3.68 **C**

Postpartum haemorrhage following a twin delivery, is likely to be due to a large placental site, and a large, over-stretched uterus which may not contract quite so efficiently immediately after delivery. Although poor placental function can occur with multiple pregnancy (particularly if it is complicated by pre-eclampsia) it is by no means universal.

3.69 **A**

3.70 **C**

Fetal blood sampling may well be able to confirm fetal distress, but the fetal blood pH will be *lower* than normal, the danger zone being below 7.20

3.71 **A**

3.72 **A**

3.73 Premature labour is common in twin pregnancy
because
the uterus is over-distended and early rupture of the membranes occurs more readily.

(*answers overleaf*)

3.73 A

SECTION VI
COMPLETION ITEMS Questions 3.74–3.93

Complete the following sentences with the appropriate word(s).

3.74 **Normal uterine contractions tend to commence from the_______________of the uterus and spread downwards through the upper and lower segments to the_______________. During this process, the contractions diminish in strength, and this gradient of tone is known as_______________. This, together with the unique property of the uterine muscle called_______________, enables muscle fibres to be drawn up and retained in the upper segment, thus leading to cervical dilatation.**

3.75 **Vaginal examination should be performed when the membranes rupture to exclude or confirm_______________.**

3.76 **Following completion of the third stage, the mother should be observed in the labour ward for at least_______________.**

3.77 **When the placenta separates centrally, it is known as a_______________separation, and if it separates from the edge initially, this is known as_______________separation.**

3.78 **Intramuscular Syntometrine 1 ml contains_______________ and_______________. It is frequently given with the birth of_______________as part of an actively managed third stage.**

3.79 **Labour may be accelerated if progress is_______________, provided there is no evidence of moderate or severe_______________.**
Prolonged labour may be due to abnormal uterine action, either hypotonic or_______________, the latter often associated with an_______________pelvis. Acceleration is most commonly achieved by the use of intravenous_______________, and the midwife must watch for signs of_______________ and_______________.

3.80 **Prolonged labour is comparatively rare in multiparous women, and may be due to_______________ labour.**

(*answers overleaf*)

3.74 a Cornua
b Cervix
c Polarity
d Retraction

3.75 Cord prolapse

3.76 One hour

3.77 a Schültze
b Matthews-Duncan

3.78 a Ergometrine 0.5 mg
b Syntocinon 5 units
c Anterior shoulder (or crowning of the head)

3.79 a Slow/delayed
b Cephalo-pelvic disproportion
c incoordinate
d android
e 'Syntocinon'
f fetal distress (hypoxia)
g tonic uterine contractions

3.80 Obstructed (labour)
Therefore i.v. Syntocinon must be used with great care, lest uterine rupture occur.

Figure 11

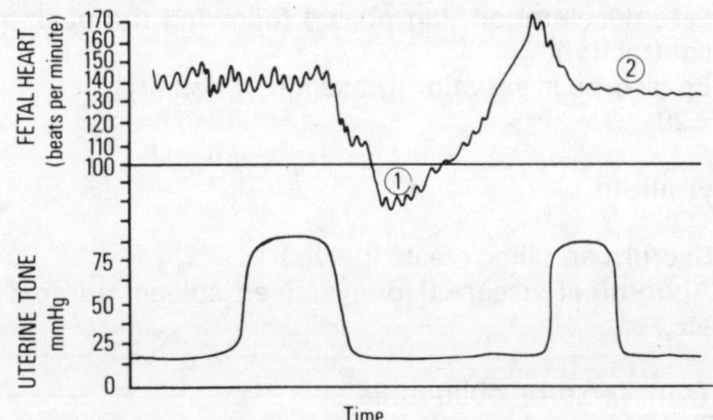

3.81 **This diagram represents part of a tracing from a___________________. The abnormal trace marked (1) is usually referred to as a___________________dip. The significant feature of this type of dip is the______________. A second abnormality is represented at (2), which shows a reduction in___________________. If the pattern marked (1) was continued, a fetal blood scalp sample might be taken. This would confirm significant fetal distress if the pH was below___________________.**

3.82 **A constriction ring may be relieved by administration of a general anaesthetic, sometimes combined with the inhalation of the drug___________________.**

3.83 **During breech delivery, the fetus should be grasped by the___________________to avoid damage to the___________________.**

3.84 **Generally, external version should only be attempted by a midwife when there is a___________________or ___________________lie with the second___________________, and no doctor is immediately available.**

3.85 **When delivering the aftercoming head of a breech, it is important to deliver the face___________________, and the vault___________________, so that sudden decompression of the head is reduced to a minimum. This will help to avoid injury, and allow the airways to be cleared.**

(*answers overleaf*)

3.81 a Cardiotocograph
b Type II (lag type) dip (or late deceleration)
c Late deceleration (lag phase) following the peak of the contraction
d Beat-to-beat variation (Baseline variability)
e 7.20

3.82 Amyl nitrite

3.83 a Sacrum and iliac crests (pelvis)
b Abdominal viscera (kidneys, liver, spleen, adrenal glands etc.)

3.84 a Transverse or oblique lie
b Twin

The other situation where a midwife might be justified in attempting external version is when a woman with an unstable lie ruptures her membranes and no medical help is immediately available.

When attempting external version the midwife must remember to make the fetus 'follow its nose', so that *flexion* will occur, and aim to achieve a *longitudinal lie* rather than a cephalic presentation.

3.85 a Quickly
b Slowly

3.86 ________________ **of the cervix, is a rare condition usually associated with very strong contractions, and a rigid cervix in a primigravida.**

3.87 **Occasionally, when one twin has died in early pregnancy, one normal, mature baby is delivered, and a** ________________ ________________ **is found, usually with the placenta.**

3.88 **Central venous pressure can be recorded from the atria, or more generally the** ________________.

3.89 **Central venous pressure indicates the amount of blood returning to the** ________________.

3.90 **The five possible outcomes of an established labour with the fetus in the occipito-posterior position are:**

a ________________
b ________________
c ________________
d ________________
e ________________.

3.91 **A patient whose blood pressure suddenly falls during surgical induction of labour, is commonly suffering from** ________________ ________________ **which may be quickly corrected by** ________________ ________________.

3.92 **The use of 'Fortral' (pentazocine) and 'Narcan Neonatal' (naloxone) by midwives is controlled by the** ________________ **Act which was made law in** ________________.

3.93 **i.v. 'Syntocinon' may be administered to induce labour, or during labour to** ________________ **it, particularly if there is** ________________ **uterine action.**

(*answers overleaf*)

3.86 Annular detachment

3.87 Fetus papyraceous (a small, flattened 'mummified' fetus)

3.88 Superior vena cava

3.89 Heart

3.90
- a Long rotation to occipito-anterior position
- b Short rotation to persistent occipito-posterior position
- c Deep transverse arrest
- d Brow presentation
- e Face presentation

3.91
- a Caval compression (supine hypotension)
- b Turning the patient onto her side, or semi-prone

3.92
- a Medicines Act
- b 1968

3.93
- a accelerate
- b hypotonic

LABOUR

The following questions are taken from recent examination papers set by the English National Board.

1. Essay questions (These answers are allocated 45 minutes)

How would a midwife recognise that labour is progressing normally? (1983)

What would lead you to suspect a breech presentation? Outline the dangers associated with a breech delivery. Describe in detail how you would deliver the after-coming head. (1983)

How would you diagnose an occipito-posterior position in labour? Discuss the possible courses of labour and their outcome. (1983)

Outline the factors influencing progress in labour. Describe in detail how the midwife assesses progress in the first stage of labour. (1983)

Women should have the right to choose where they will be confined and the total management they receive. Discuss this statement with particular emphasis on labour and delivery. (1983)

Discuss the responsibilities of the midwife when caring for a woman in labour. (1983)

Outline the factors that put the fetus at risk during labour. How may fetal distress be recognised and managed? (1983)

Discuss your management of the admission of a primigravida in early labour. How would you help her husband to become involved in her subsequent care? (1983)

Describe the methods of pain relief available to women in labour. What factors could influence the choice? (1983)

Mrs Green, a 23-year-old primigravida who is 42 weeks pregnant, is admitted to a consultant unit for induction of labour by amniotomy and intravenous oxytocin. How should the midwife prepare Mrs Green for these procedures? Describe the care given until labour is established. (1984)

A twin pregnancy has been diagnosed in a multigravid woman. Labour commences spontaneously at 38 weeks gestation. Describe the management of the second and third stages of this labour. List the complications which may occur. (1984)

Explain in detail your management of the third stage of labour, and outline the complications which may occur. (1984)

List the factors responsible for delay in the first stage of labour. How may the midwife recognise this delay? What should be her management? (1984)

How can the midwife meet the individual needs of the woman and her partner throughout labour? (1984)

How does a midwife recognise and monitor normal progress in the second stage of labour? What preparations should a midwife make for a safe delivery? (1984)

List the indications for a vaginal examination to be performed by a midwife during labour.
What information can a midwife obtain from this examination? (1984)

In accordance with the Midwives Rules the midwife is required to keep detailed records of all cases she attends.
What records are kept during pregnancy and labour?
Discuss the need for and the significance of these records. (1984)

Describe normal and abnormal fetal heart patterns during labour. How may the midwife recognise fetal distress:
a. In the home?
b. In a well-equipped delivery suite? (1985)

Define postpartum haemorrhage.
List the factors which pre-dispose to primary postpartum haemorrhage and discuss its prevention and management. (1985)

2. Write briefly on each of the following subjects:
Observations on a woman receiving epidural anaesthesia during labour (1983)
Ketosis in labour (1983)
The midwife's responsibility concerning the placenta and membranes following delivery (1983)
Pain relief in labour (1983)
Indications for performing an episiotomy (1983)
Delivery of the shoulders (1983)
Pre-disposing factors of primary postpartum haemorrhage (1983)
Causes of premature rupture of membranes (1983)
Use of oxytocic drugs in labour (1983)
Causes of maternal hypotension in labour (1983)
Preparing a woman for caesarean section (1983)
Artificial rupture of membranes (1983)
Signs of uterine rupture in labour (1983)
Deep transverse arrest of the fetal head (1983)
Influence of an anthropoid pelvis on labour (1983)

Inhalational analgesia (1983)
Records made by the midwife during the second stage of labour (1983)
The importance of fluid balance in labour (1983)
Shoulder dystocia (1983)
Acceleration of the first stage of labour (1983)
Advantages of a well-flexed head in labour (1984)
Abnormalities of amniotic fluid in labour (1984)
Positions of a mother for delivery (1984)
Prevention of perineal damage (1984)
A research study/ report concerned with a midwifery aspect of labour (1984)
Constituents and effects of 'syntometrine' (1984)
Clinical evidence of full dilatation of the cervical os (1984)
Protection of a woman's privacy during labour (1984)
Procedure for identification of the mother and baby including the details required (1984)
Use of pethidine in labour (1984)
Principles of perineal repair (1984)
Fetal well-being in the second stage of labour (1984)
Entonox (1984)
Methods of delivery of the placenta (1984)
Causes of a retained placenta (1985)
Mendelson's syndrome (1985)
Birth plans (1985)
Meconium stained liquor (1985)
Face presentation (1985)
Perineal shaving (1985)

4. Postnatal period and family planning

SECTION I
SINGLE RESPONSE MULTIPLE CHOICE QUESTIONS Questions 4.1–4.28

Select a *single* correct response to each of the following questions:

4.1 The normal discharge from the uterus following childbirth is termed:
A leucorrhoea
B decidua
C lochia
D operculum

4.2 One of the physiological changes in the cardio-vascular system in the early postnatal period is:
A hypovolaemia
B hypervolaemia
C haemodilution
D haemoconcentration

4.3 A positive Homan's sign may indicate:
A deep vein thrombosis
B pulmonary embolism
C a low prothrombin level
D thrombocytopenia

4.4 Pulmonary embolism is commonly associated with:
A thrombophlebitis
B phlebothrombosis
C Christmas disease
D a low prothrombin level

(*answers overleaf*)

4.1 **C**

Lochia is the discharge from the uterus—chiefly the placental site—containing blood, decidua, leucocytes, etc. It persists in decreasing amount for 1–2 weeks following childbirth. Leucorrhoea is the increased secretion of cervical mucus which often occurs in pregnancy.

4.2 **D**

Haemodilution occurs during pregnancy when the blood volume increases, and is *reversed* following a marked diuresis after delivery. Hypovolaemia and hypervolaemia are pathological conditions possibly indicating severe haemorrhage or overtransfusion respectively.

4.3 **A**

If a deep vein thrombosis is present in the lower limb, sharp dorsiflexion of the foot towards the shin will generally elicit distinct pain in the calf of the affected leg. This is a positive Homan's sign, but it should be elicited with care, as carried out too forcefully can cause a clot to be dislodged, and so lead to pulmonary embolus.

4.4 **B**

In thrombophlebitis the vein wall is inflamed, and any clot formation usually firmly adherent. However, a phlebothrombosis generally occurs in the larger veins, and the clot is easily detached within the vessel, and may produce an embolus.

4.5 Secondary postpartum haemorrhage is most likely to occur in the postnatal period during:

A day 1–3
B day 4–6
C day 10–14
D day 14–21

4.6 When rubella immunisation is given to postnatal mothers, efficient contraceptive measures must be taken for a minimum of:

A 1 month
B 3 months
C 6 months
D 9 months

4.7 The Kleihauer test is performed to detect:

A rhesus antibodies
B rubella antibodies
C fetal cells
D human chorionic gonadotrophin

4.8 When discussing the most effective method of contraception, the final decision should be made by:

A the general practitioner
B the client
C the clinic doctor
D the nurse

4.9 Coitus interruptus is a term used to describe:

A premature ejaculation
B withdrawal before ejaculation
C the 'safe' period
D a test for infertility

4.10 Menarche is a term implying:

A age at first menstruation
B the climacteric
C a disorder of menstruation
D a menopausal symptom

4.11 The *highest* recommended dose of oestrogen to be contained in any contraceptive pill is:

A 30 micrograms
B 50 micrograms
C 20 micrograms
D 70 micrograms

(*answers overleaf*)

4.5 **C**
Commonly associated with retained, infected fragments of placenta or membranes.

4.6 **B**
If conception occurs in the three months following rubella immunisation, there is a very high risk of congenital abnormality for the fetus. It is therefore imperative that a very effective method of contraception is used during this period e.g. combined oestrogen/progestogen 'pill', or when client motivation is suspect, an intra-uterine contraceptive device or progestogen injection e.g. 'Depo-Provera'.

4.7 **C**
The test differentiates between fetal and adult haemoglobin, and is used to assess the magnitude of feto-maternal haemorrhage in rhesus negative women, so that the correct dose of anti-D immunoglobulin can be given to the mother.

4.8 **B**
Advice can be offered, but the client must always make the final decision.

4.9 **B**
This is a widely used, but unreliable method of contraception.

4.10 **A**

4.11 **B**
Many brands of the combined 'pill' now have considerably less oestrogen content:
e.g. Microgynon 30 (30 micrograms)
Loestrin (20 micrograms)

4.12 What is the maximum time lapse to take a forgotten combined oestrogen/progestogen contraceptive pill:
A four hours
B eight hours
C eighteen hours
D twenty-four hours

4.13 'Progestogen only' oral contraceptives are usually prescribed for:
A postmenopausal women
B diabetic women
C mothers who are breast-feeding
D women with a history of menorrhagia

4.14 Oral contraception using the combined oestrogen/progestogen 'pill' is contra-indicated in women with a history of:
A pyelonephritis
B phenylketonuria
C cholecystitis
D thrombo-embolic disease

4.15 Spermicides remain active for a maximum time of:
A two hours
B three hours
C six hours
D eight hours

4.16 The most suitable intra-uterine device for a nullipara is:
A Dalkon shield
B Lippes loop
C Saf-T coil
D Copper 7

4.17 Dyspareunia is a term used to describe:
A a scrotal infection
B menstrual pain
C sterility
D painful coitus

4.18 When a cervical smear is taken at a clinic, the general practitioner should be informed:
A if a positive result is obtained
B if a negative result is obtained
C if an infection is present
D on every occasion

(*answers overleaf*)

4.12 **B**
If more than eight hours has elapsed, the client should be advised to take the missed pill, and then continue taking the 'pill' as normal, but to take additional precautions (e.g. sheath) until the end of the cycle. This is of particular importance with 'pills' containing a low dose of oestrogen i.e. <50 micrograms.

4.13 **C**
This form of oral contraception is slightly less reliable than the combined 'pill'. The progestogens act on the cervical mucus, making it thick, hostile and impenetrable to the sperm. Its advantage lies in the fact that it does not diminish lactation.

4.14 **D**
There is a proven link between oestrogens and thrombo-embolic disease, particularly where other predisposing factors exist, e.g. varicose veins.

4.15 **B**
Additional spermicidal cream/foam/jelly should be used if intercourse is to take place after three to four hours.

4.16 **D**
The small Copper 7 (Minigravigard) has the smallest introducer, which can pass through the cervix in women who has never borne children. However, some doctors still use other intrauterine contraceptive devices including the Nova-T.

4.17 **D**

4.18 **D**

4.19 A cervical smear should be taken from:
A the cervical os
B the anterior fornix
C the posterior fornix
D the cervical canal

4.20 Dyskaryosis is a term used to describe:
A an abnormality of cervical cytology
B a cervical erosion
C a vaginal infection
D presence of cervical malignancy

4.21 Vasectomy is effective:
A immediately
B after three months
C after two clear sperm counts
D after thirty ejaculations

4.22 Female sterilisation is effective:
A immediately
B following dilatation and curettage
C after three months
D after six months

4.23 A motile protozoan is the causative organism of:
A gonorrhoea
B trichomonas vaginitis
C vaginal candidiasis
D syphilis

4.24 Nystatin is the drug used to treat:
A candidiasis
B trichomoniasis
C genital warts
D non-specific cervicitis

4.25 A multigravid patient suddenly develops oedema, epigastric pain, and hypertension 24 hours following a normal delivery. Would you suspect the onset of:
A sub-arachnoid haemorrhage
B eclampsia
C cardiac failure
D essential hypertension

(*answers overleaf*)

4.19 **A**
The external cervical os contains the squamo-columnar epithelial junction, which is particularly prone to initial malignant change.

4.20 **A**
Dyskaryosis does not inevitably indicate a carcinoma *in situ*, but it shows cell abnormality, and must be further investigated, e.g. by repeat smear, and/or cervical biopsy.

4.21 **C**
These two clear sperm counts should be at least one month apart.

4.22 **A**
Female sterilisation is usually carried out early in the postnatal period, or prior to ovulation, and is therefore considered to be effective at once.

4.23 **B**
The common treatment for trichomoniasis is metronidazole (Flagyl) 200 mg t.d.s. for 7–10 days. The sexual partner may also require treatment.

4.24 **A**
This drug is usually prescribed in the form of pessaries or cream, and must be used, as directed, for *at least* 14 days if the infection is not to recur. The sexual partner may need a course of oral Nystatin if he is a reservoir of infection.

4.25 **B**
Postpartum eclampsia occurs in 20–30 per cent of all cases of eclampsia. It often presents suddenly, with few warning signs, and almost always within 48 hours of delivery.

CASE HISTORY

A 40-year-old multipara from a low income family is two days postpartum, and about to return home from the maternity hospital. She is breast-feeding her baby, and she has a history of thrombophlebitis.

Using the above information, answer the three questions which follow:

4.26 Which of the following problems are particularly likely to affect this baby?

A diabetes insipidus
B sarcoma
C Down's syndrome
D haemangioma

4.27 If breast-feeding continues for many months, which of the following complications could ensue in the mother?

A iron-deficiency anaemia
B thalassaemia
C influenza
D toxoplasmosis

4.28 This mother is anxious not to conceive again, as she now has five children. Which would be the most effective and suitable method of contraception for her?

A safe period
B sheath
C contraceptive pill
D sterilisation

(*answers overleaf*)

4.26 **C**

Down's syndrome (Trisomy 21) becomes increasingly common in mothers over 40 years.

4.27 **A**

The mother with several children in a low income family may well commence her pregnancy with depleted iron stores. She also tends to have a poor diet, which combined with long-term breast-feeding, may reduce her haemoglobin level still further. Women who eat a well-balanced diet, and have well-spaced pregnancies, are unlikely to become anaemic just because they are breast-feeding, as breast-milk contains only small quantities of iron.

4.28 **D**

The so called 'safe period' is generally an unreliable method with a high failure rate, and the best results need great application on the part of the woman. Equally, the sheath (condom) requires excellent motivation from the male partner. The progestogen-only 'pill' is less reliable than the combined oestrogen-progestogen 'pill', and the latter is contra-indicated due to her age and history of thrombophlebitis. At 40, and with an established family, sterilisation, if acceptable to both parents, would seem to be indicated.

SECTION II

MULTIPLE RESPONSE QUESTIONS Questions 4.29–4.42
Select any number of correct responses between 1–5.

4.29 Postnatal exercises can lead to:
A the return of tone to the levator ani muscles
B subinvolution of the uterus
C frequency of micturition
D an improvement in transient stress incontinence
E an increase in abdominal muscle tone

4.30 Lactation:
A is stimulated by the baby suckling
B can be reduced by severe infection or emotional trauma
C is associated with high levels of prolactin
D involves the secretion of milk in the alveoli of the breast
E is preceded by the production of colostrum

4.31 In the early postnatal period:
A the lochia normally increases in amount
B the mother's mood may be depressed and unstable
C a poor diuresis occurs during the first few days
D the uterus will steadily decrease in size
E it is usual for the pulse rate to rise significantly

4.32 Secondary postpartum haemorrhage:
A is often caused by infected, retained products of conception
B occurs mainly in primigravid women
C is usually associated with vasa praevia
D can be associated with a succenturiate placenta
E tends to occur around the 10th–14th day postpartum

4.33 Which of the following would cause you to suspect a *serious* psychosis in the early postnatal period:
A tearfulness
B hallucinations
C mild depression
D persistent insomnia
E excessive thirst

4.34 Heparin:
A crosses the placenta
B is found in large quantities in the amniotic fluid
C has its action reversed by protamine sulphate
D acts as an anticoagulant
E is usually given intramuscularly

(*answers overleaf*)

4.29 **A D E**

4.30 **A B C D E**

4.31 **B D**
During the first week of the puerperium, the lochia normally *decreases* in amount; there is a marked diuresis, and the pulse rate usually falls, following the exertions of labour.

4.32 **A D E**

4.33 **B D**
Visual or auditory hallucinations, and intractable insomnia, should always be treated as possible warning signs of an impending psychosis, while tearfulness and mild depression may be part of the physiological emotional upheaval which follows most pregnancies.

4.34 **C D**
Heparin is most commonly administered by the intravenous route, and does not cross the placenta to the fetus. It is, therefore, the anticoagulant of choice in pregnancy.

4.35 When using Milton or a similar hypochlorite sterilising agent for feeding utensils:
- **A** The solution must be changed every 24 hours
- **B** the utensils should be rinsed before use
- **C** metal articles should not be immersed in this solution
- **D** it is important to exclude all air from utensils when immersed
- **E** utensils do not need to be cleansed prior to immersion

4.36 Breast infection is often associated with:
- **A** a flushed breast
- **B** inverted nipple
- **C** staphylococcus aureus
- **D** cracked nipple
- **E** postpartum eclampsia

4.37 Organisms commonly associated with infection of the female urinary tract include:
- **A** Döderlein's bacilli
- **B** escherichia coli
- **C** treponema pallidum
- **D** bacillus proteus
- **E** salmonella

4.38 Mothers should take their babies regularly to the child health clinic:
- **A** to be weighed
- **B** to have their development assessed
- **C** to have sight and hearing tested
- **D** if they have an infection
- **E** for advice on feeding and child care

4.39 Insomnia in the postnatal period may indicate:
- **A** sore perineum
- **B** puerperal psychosis
- **C** lochia serosa
- **D** overfull breasts
- **E** a retroverted uterus

4.40 If the fundal height appears to be at the level of the umbilicus on the fourth day following a normal delivery, the cause could be:
- **A** lochia alba
- **B** intra-uterine infection
- **C** over-distention of the bladder
- **D** ischio-rectal haematoma
- **E** retained membranes or placenta

(*answers overleaf*)

4.35 **A B C D**
All articles should be scrupulously clean *before* immersion. Most manufacturers recommend that at home parents do rinse equipment with cooled boiled water before use. However in maternity hospitals because of the added infection risk, rinsing may *not* be carried out.

4.36 **A C D**
Staphylococcus aureus is probably the most common causative organism in breast infections.

4.37 **B D**

4.38 **A B C E**
Ill children should be taken to the general practitioner, and not allowed to put children who are well at risk.

4.39 **A B D**
Remember that a sore perineum or tender breasts are a more common cause of insomnia than a psychosis!

4.40 **B C E**
A full bladder may well simulate a bulky uterus, and by the fourth postpartum day, the problem may well be retention with overflow, which will need prompt treatment to restore normal bladder tone and function.

4.41 Early ambulation following childbirth:

A is essential following epidural analgesia
B helps to reduce the incidence of deep vein thrombosis
C increases autolysis
D assists efficient emptying of the bladder
E predisposes to perineal sepsis

4.42 At the six week postnatal examination, the doctor will routinely carry out:

A pelvic examination
B breast examination
C blood pressure
D Homan's test
E Kleihauer test

(*answers overleaf*)

4.41 **B D**
Following epidural analgesia, if the mother cannot be mobilised within a few hours of delivery, it is important to encourage both active and passive leg exercises.

4.42 **A B C**

SECTION III
TRUE OR FALSE? Questions 4.43–4.52

Indicate whether you think the statements listed below are true or false.

4.43 **Mothers should be encouraged to attend for a postnatal check-up six weeks after delivery.**

4.44 **Amniotic fluid embolism may lead to severe coagulation disorders.**

4.45 **Depression in the early postnatal period is due to the sudden rise in progesterone levels.**

4.46 **It is usual for the fully breast-fed baby to gain 60–90 g in weight in the initial 2–3 days of life.**

4.47 **Placental site infection, if neglected, can lead to salpingitis and subsequent infertility.**

4.48 **'Afterpains' in breast-feeding mothers are caused by the production of prolactin during feeding.**

4.49 **Vulval or ischio-rectal haematoma formation can be a painful aftermath of a difficult delivery.**

4.50 **Mastitis or breast abscess formation rarely occur prior to the eighth postnatal day, and are more common in the 2nd–4th week.**

4.51 **Incontinence of urine can be due to vesico-vaginal fistula.**

4.52 **Postnatal exercises will strengthen the pelvic floor, and help to prevent uterine prolapse in later life.**

(*answers overleaf*)

4.43 **True**

4.44 **True**
This may be hypofibrinogenaemia, or a more profound disseminated intravascular coagulation.

4.45 **False**
Progesterone levels *fall* in the early postnatal period, following the expulsion of the placenta.

4.46 **False**
The fully breast-fed baby generally loses a small amount of weight in the first few days of life, but should be gaining steadily, and back to his birth weight by the 10th day.

4.47 **True**

4.48 **False**
'Afterpains' are caused by the increased production of oxytocin, which is stimulated by the baby suckling. Oxytocin contracts the uterine muscle, and may produce a pain rather like dysmenorrhoea.

4.49 **True**
A considerable amount of blood may be lost, and the haematoma may have to be evacuated, and the bleeding point ligated. The patient may be shocked and require a blood transfusion.

4.50 **True**

4.51 **True**

4.52 **True**

SECTION IV
MATCHING ITEMS Questions 4.53–4.56

Match the items in Group 1 with the most appropriate item in Group 2. (Each item in Group 2 may only be used *once*.)

4.53 Match the items in Group 1 with the most appropriate item in Group 2.

Group 1
- **(i)** subinvolution
- **(ii)** cervical smear
- **(iii)** third degree tear
- **(iv)** artificial feeding

Group 2
- **A** overweight babies
- **B** carcinoma *in situ*
- **C** retained products of conception
- **D** perineal pain
- **E** Heminevrin therapy

4.54 Match the items in Group 1 with the most appropriate item in Group 2.

Group 1
- **(i)** inverted nipples
- **(ii)** retention of urine
- **(iii)** vesico-vaginal fistula
- **(iv)** puerperal pyrexia

Group 2
- **A** breast feeding
- **B** intra-uterine infection
- **C** epidural analgesia
- **D** Woolwich shells
- **E** difficult forceps delivery

4.55 Match the drugs in Group 1 with the condition they are most commonly used to treat in Group 2.

Group 1
- **(i)** quinestrol ('Estrovis')
- **(ii)** ergometrine tablets
- **(iii)** paracetamol
- **(iv)** methyldopa ('Aldomet')

Group 2
- **A** hypertension
- **B** puerperal depression
- **C** suppression of lactation
- **D** retained membranes
- **E** afterpains

4.56 Match the hormones in Group 1 with the most appropriate action from Group 2.

Group 1
- **(i)** prolactin
- **(ii)** oestrogen
- **(iii)** progesterone
- **(iv)** oxytocin

Group 2
- **A** stimulates production of milk producing tissue
- **B** stimulates milk ejection
- **C** stimulates milk production
- **D** stimulates the corpus luteum
- **E** stimulates the growth of the duct system in the breast

(*answers overleaf*)

4.53

(i) **C**
(ii) **B**
(iii) **D**
(iv) **A**

4.54

(i) **D**
(ii) **C**
(iii) **E**
(iv) **B**

4.55

(i) **C**
(ii) **D**
(iii) **E**
(iv) **A**

4.56

(i) **C**
(ii) **E**
(iii) **A**
(iv) **B**

SECTION V
ASSERTION/REASON Questions 4.57–4.60

Read carefully the five possible answers listed below marked A, B, C, D and E. Select which is appropriate for the assertions and reasons which follow.

A Assertion true; reason is a true statement and is the correct reason.
B Assertion and reason both true, but reason is *not* the correct reason.
C Assertion is true, but reason is a false statement.
D Assertion is false, but the reason is a true statement.
E Assertion and reason are both false.

4.57 **Urinary tract infection is a common cause of puerperal pyrexia**
because
a significant diuresis occurs immediately following delivery.

4.58 **Breast feeding is best for all infants**
because
there is a reduced risk of overfeeding and hypernatraemia.

4.59 **In the early postnatal period, urinary tract infection is common**
because
the bladder and urethra have been bruised during labour, and the bladder is frequently atonic following the delivery.

4.60 **Breast feeding is recommended to most mothers**
because
there is a reduced infection risk to the baby in the first months of life.

(*answers overleaf*)

4.57 **B**
Both statements are true, but do not relate to each other.

4.58 **D**
Breast feeding is usually best for most normal infants, but is contraindicated in conditions such as galactosaemia, where the baby cannot tolerate the galactose in breast milk.

4.59 **A**

4.60 **A**

SECTION VI
COMPLETION ITEMS Questions 4.61–4.70

Supply the missing word(s) in the following statements:

4.61 **Oxytocin is produced by the_______________gland and acts on the_______________cells in the breast, which pump the milk from the alveoli through the lactiferous tubules.**

4.62 **Involution is caused by the enzymatic digestion of excess uterine muscle. This process is known as_______________, the metabolic waste products from this process are excreted through the kidneys, and may be manifest in a raised blood_______________.**

4.63 **Postpartum sterilisation is best carried out within 3–4 days of delivery, because _______________.**

4.64 **There is usually an initial weight loss in the early postnatal period as excess_______________is eliminated, and blood volume stabilises. Following this some body fat is generally lost, especially when the mother_______________ her baby.**

4.65 **Eclampsia is a rare complication in the puerperium, and normally occurs within_______________hours of delivery.**

4.66 **If the mother decides to bottle feed her baby, it is best to suppress lactation by supporting the breasts efficiently, and giving mild analgesia as needed._______________ should be avoided, they may predispose to deep vein thrombosis.**

4.67 **Breast milk contains less protein than cow's milk, and this protein consists mainly of the easily digestible_______________ and a smaller percentage of_______________, which tends to form indigestible curds.**

4.68 **Following childbirth, the cervix has a slit-like opening which is sometimes referred to as a_______________.**

4.69 **Severe postpartum haemorrhage can leave the woman with Sheehan's syndrome, which is caused by_______________.**

4.70 **The primary stimulus to lactation is_______________.**

(*answers overleaf*)

4.61 a Posterior pituitary
b Myo-epithelial cells

4.62 a Autolysis
b Urea

4.63 The uterus and tubes are still *abdominal* organs, and therefore easily accessible to the surgeon. However, it is most important that the baby is found to be fit, and that the parents receive effective counselling before such a decision is made.

4.64 a Body fluid
b Breast feeds

4.65 48 hours

4.66 Oestrogens

4.67 a Lactalbumin
b Caseinogen

4.68 'Multip's os'

4.69 An ischaemic necrosis of the pituitary gland

4.70 Suckling
The mechanical compression of the nipple and deep aveolar tissues by the jaws of the baby initiates a neuro-hormonal reflex between the pituitary gland and the hypothalamus. The *anterior* pituitary gland responds by secreting prolactin, which causes the acini cells in the alveoli to produce milk. At the same time, the *posterior* pituitary gland secretes oxytocin, which stimulates the contractile myo-epithelial cells surrounding the alveoli and lactiferous ducts, thus pumping milk along the duct system to the nipple area.

POSTNATAL PERIOD AND FAMILY PLANNING

The following questions are taken from recent examination papers set by the English National Board.

1. Essay questions (These questions are allocated 45 minutes)

What is the role of the midwife in relation to a mother and her baby during the puerperium? For what reasons may liaison with other personnel and services be required? (1983)

A mother 48-hours after delivery has a raised temperature. List the possible causes of the pyrexia, and describe the midwife's care of this woman. (1983)

What do you understand by the term puerperal psychosis? What may be the predisposing causes?
How may the midwife recognise the onset of this condition? (1983)

Outline the arrangements that have to be made for a planned early transfer home. What problems affecting the mother may the community midwife encounter and how should she deal with them? (1983)

Discuss the responsibilities of the midwife in the care of a mother and baby who is delivered by caesarean section. (1983)

Discuss the role of the midwife in assisting parents in their choice of contraceptive methods. (1983)

Some mothers are dismayed by their lack of maternal feeling following the birth of their baby. What contributory factors may give rise to this situation?
How may the midwife assist in allaying the mother's feelings of inadequacy and improve the mother/baby relationship? (1983)

Describe the predisposing causes of deep vein thrombosis in women during the postnatal period.
How may this condition be recognised and treated? (1983)

Discuss the help and advice a midwife should give to parents to assist in the establishment of infant feeding (1983)

Some women on a postnatal ward are unlikely to receive the care and support they need. Why may this be so?
How could the situation be improved? (1983)

What problems of micturition may a woman experience during the postnatal period? Describe the prevention and management of these disorders. (1983)

**Each mother and baby has individual needs.
How does the midwife recognise and meet these needs in the postnatal period? (1984)**

What assistance can a midwife give to a mother who has already decided on the method of feeding her baby? (1984)

**A mother and her baby are to be transferred home from hospital on the third day following delivery.
How should the midwife prepare the mother for this event and what information should the community midwife receive? (1984)**

Mrs Jones is transferred from the labour ward, having had a difficult forceps delivery and her baby admitted to the Special Care Baby Unit. What care and support should the midwife give to the mother during the first 24 hours in the postnatal ward? (1984)

**A mother has a secondary postpartum haemorrhage on the ninth day. List the possible causes.
Describe your management of this condition in the woman's home. (1984)**

**A newly delivered mother is considering offering her baby for adoption. Describe the special skills required of the midwife.
What knowledge of other services will help the midwife to meet the total needs of this woman? (1984)**

**Postnatal care can be provided in several ways following a hospital based delivery.
Discuss the alternatives available.
How should the midwife assist the family in making their choice? (1984)**

**Describe the changes in mood and varying degrees of depression in a mother in the postnatal period.
In what ways may a midwife assist the mother during this time?
How would she recognise when other specialist help is required? (1984)**

What factors may influence the choice of contraception for a woman and her partner following the birth of their first baby? (1984)

Mrs Hughes has just been admitted to a postnatal ward following delivery of a severely abnormal baby which is not expected to live. Describe the role of the midwife in this situation. (1984)

Describe how the midwife assists a woman to gain confidence and competence in her new role as a mother during the postnatal period. (1984)

**Describe in detail the physiological process of involution.
How may the midwife recognise this clinically?
What might be her management when involution is delayed. (1984)**

A young primigrivida has been delivered of a stillborn infant:
a. What are the statutory duties of the midwife?
b. How may the midwife contribute to the emotional support of the bereaved parents?
c. How may the parents be counselled about future pregnancies? (1985)

**What are the advantages and disadvantages of remaining in hospital for six days after a normal delivery?
How can a midwife make this stay a happy experience for the new mother and her family? (1985)**

**A mother has a difficult forceps delivery.
List the main complications which may occur.
Describe the midwifery care and management of this mother in the first week following delivery. (1985)**

2. **Write briefly on each of the following subjects:**
Importance of postnatal examination 6 weeks after the birth (1983)
Problems of a mother with language difficulties (1983)
Role of the father in the postnatal period (1983)
Purpose of postnatal exercises (1983)
Pre-disposing factors of deep vein thrombosis (1983)
Administration of Anti-D gamma globulin (1983)
Main causes of maternal mortality (1983)
Retention of urine following delivery (1983)
Importance of early ambulation following delivery (1983)
Secondary postpartum haemorrhage (1983)
Postnatal depression (1983)
Recognition of uterine infection in the first 10 days following delivery (1983)
Perineal pain in the postnatal period (1983)
Natural family planning methods (1983)
Maternal records maintained by the midwife (1983)
Sore nipples (1983)
'Rooming in' (1983)
Effects on the woman of perineal suturing (1983)
Vaginal haematoma (1984)
Investigation of raised maternal temperature (1984)
Postnatal problems associated with epidural anaesthesia during labour (1984)
Postnatal support groups (1984)
Sub-involution of the uterus (1984)
Difficulties with sexual intercourse when the woman has had a perineal repair (1984)

Prolonged separation of the mother from her baby (1984)
A research study/report concerned with the postnatal period (1984)
Value of postnatal exercises (1984)
Abdominal examination on the third day (1984)
Statutory duties of a midwife during the postnatal period (1984)
Promotion of rest and sleep in a postnatal ward (1984)
The midwifery process (1984)
Stress incontinence (1985)
Recognition of postnatal depression (1985)
Hormonal contraception (1985)
Role of the father in the postnatal period (1985)
Suppression of lactation (1985)
Vulval haematoma (1985)
Retention of urine (1985)
Kleihauer test (1985)
Causes of subinvolution of the uterus (1985)

5. Neonatal paediatrics

SECTION I
SINGLE RESPONSE MULTIPLE CHOICE QUESTIONS Questions 5.1–5.24

Select a *single* correct response to each of the following questions:

5.1 The test for congenital dislocation of the hip is:
A Apgar
B Ortolani
C Silverman
D Bishop

5.2 The major part of the protein content of cow's milk is:
A lactose
B caseinogen
C lactogen
D lactalbumin

5.3 Breast engorgement in the neonate is due to the alterations in hormone balance, and can be seen in both males and females. It should be treated by:
A aspiration
B expression
C masterly inactivity
D antibiotic therapy

5.4 Milia:
A are small white spots on the hard palate
B are white spots sometimes present on the face of the newborn
C appear on the tongue when a baby has thrush
D appear on the buttocks in nappy rash

(*answers overleaf*)

5.1 **B**

Both Ortolani and Barlow devised similar tests, to screen newborn babies for congenital dislocation of the hip.

5.2 **B**

In cow's milk the protein content is 3.5 per cent of which 3 per cent is caseinogen, and only 0.5 per cent the more digestible lactalbumin. In human milk there is less total protein (1.5 per cent), but 1 per cent is lactalbumin and only 0.5 per cent caseinogen.

5.3 **C**

On no account should any attempt be made to express the engorged breast, or secondary infection may intervene. If left well alone it will subside within a few days.

5.4 **B**

Milia should not be touched—they last only a few weeks.

5.5 The umbilical cord stump normally separates by a process of:
A nidation
B fibrosis
C dry gangrene
D autolysis

5.6 In the neonate, a hairy mole at the base of the spine may indicate:
A imperforate anus
B pilonidal sinus
C Hirschsprung's disease
D occult spina bifida

5.7 Which of the following will predispose a newborn infant to intracranial haemorrhage:
A hyperbilirubinaemia
B hypoxia
C kernicterus
D hypernatraemia

5.8 Serum bilirubin 340 micromol/l is equivalent to:
A 3 mg/100 ml
B 10 mg/100 ml
C 20 mg/100 mg
D 25 mg/100 ml

5.9 At 3–4 weeks of age the pre-term infant should receive a dietary supplement of:
A potassium
B iron
C sodium
D magnesium

5.10 Death from intraventricular haemorrhage is most commonly associated with:
A breast-fed infants
B pre-term infants
C physiological jaundice
D postmature infants

5.11 Tentorial tears associated with breech delivery are due to:
A increased red cell fragility
B excessive moulding
C compression and decompression of the fetal head
D cephalhaematoma

(*answers overleaf*)

5.5 **C**

This is why it is important to keep the cord stump dry and clean. If moist infection occurs, it may slow down cord separation, and track back up the ductus venosus to the liver and systemic circulation, which can lead to septicaemia.

5.6 **D**

5.7 **B**

There is no doubt that hypoxia predisposes to, and increases the severity of intracranial bleeding in the neonate.

5.8 **C**

A useful approximation is to multiply the old milligram by 17, e.g.
20 mg × 17 = 340 micromol/l
10 mg × 17 = 170 micromol/l

5.9 **B**

Oral iron supplements are not absorbed until the infant is 3–4 weeks old.

5.10 **B**

Intraventricular haemorrhage (i.e. into the ventricles of the brain) is confined almost entirely to significantly pre-term infants.

5.11 **C**

As the fetal head is rapidly compressed and driven into the pelvis by powerful second stage contractions, it does not have time to mould, and is equally rapidly decompressed at delivery, unless very careful control is exercised by the accoucheur.

5.12 A defect in the abdominal wall through which the bowel protrudes is known as:
A myelocele
B exomphalos
C syndactyly
D hydrocele

5.13 The Sweat test is used to diagnose:
A diabetes mellitus
B hypothyroidism
C galactosaemia
D cystic fibrosis

5.14 'Narcan neonatal' (naloxone) may be used at birth, when the infant's respiratory centre has been depressed due to the use of drugs such as pethidine for maternal pain relief in labour. The safe dose for a mature infant is:
A 1 ml per kg body weight
B 0.1 mg per kg body weight
C 0.01 mg per kg body weight
D 0.5 ml per kg body weight

5.15 When measuring the blood glucose levels with 'Dextrostix', which of the following results would indicate that the infant is hypoglycaemic:
A 5.5 mmol/litre
B 5.2 mmol/litre
C 4.0 mmol/litre
D 1.2 mmol/litre

5.16 A red, excoriated ring around the anus in the neonate is likely to be due to an infection caused by:
A streptococcus faecalis
B escherichia coli
C pneumococcus
D candida albicans

5.17 If the mother ingests tetracyclines during her pregnancy, fetal damage may occur. This will manifest itself in the baby as:
A deafness
B congenital heart disease
C Mongolian blue spot
D yellow discolouration of the teeth

(answers overleaf)

5.12 **B**
Where there is a large herniation of gut with no covering peritoneal sac, it is known as a gastroschisis.

5.13 **D**
Cystic fibrosis (mucoviscidosis) is a congenital anomaly of the mucus-secreting glands throughout the body, and clinically it particularly affects the pancreas and lungs.

5.14 **C**
When using naloxone (Narcan), it is *vital* to check whether the ampoule is the adult (0.4 mg/ml), or the neonatal (0.02 mg/ml) preparation.

5.15 **D**
1.2 mmol/l = 25 mg/100 ml blood glucose.

5.16 **D**
This is indication that candidiasis has infected the whole alimentary tract, and an oral suspension of Nystatin needs to be used rather than local treatment for the mouth infection alone.

5.17 **B**
The use of this antibiotic should be avoided throughout pregnancy for this reason.

5.18 If the mother is prescribed Valium (diazepam) in late pregnancy or labour, the neonate is likely to be more difficult to resuscitate and to suffer from:

A hyperpyrexia
B muscular hypotonia
C paroxysmal tachycardia
D eczema

5.19 Hypospadias is:

A a form of polycystic kidney
B when the testicles are undescended
C when the urethra opens on the under surface of the penis
D part of the epididymis

5.20 Babies are often born with a white, greasy substance on their skin. This is called:

A lanugo
B petechiae
C vernix
D vertex

5.21 At birth the mature baby has a haemoglobin level in the region of:

A 10–12 g/dl
B 12–14 g/dl
C 16–18 g/dl
D 20–40 g/dl

5.22 Congenital cataract may be due to a maternal infection such as:

A influenza
B chickenpox
C tuberculosis
D rubella

5.23 Inability to breathe through the nose when feeding may be due to:

A choanal atresia
B oesophageal atresia
C cleft lip
E tongue tie

(*answers overleaf*)

5.18 **B**
These infants are often born with very poor muscle tone which may persist for several days, which is why many doctors prefer to avoid the use of diazepam, particularly in labour.

5.19 **C**
The other similar anomaly is epispadias, where the urethral meatus emerges somewhere on the dorsal (top) surface of penis. Both conditions need extensive plastic surgery to correct them.

5.20 **C**
This substance helps to protect the skin from the liquor amnii during intrauterine life.

5.21 **C**

5.22 **D**
The congenital rubella syndrome frequently includes congenital cataract. In can also be hereditary or be from other causes, e.g. metabolic disorders, such as galactosaemia.

5.23 **A**
Choanal atresia is a congenital blockage between the nose and the pharynx, and if bilateral will prevent the baby from sucking and breathing at the same time.
Surgical correction is usually carried out immediately, so that the baby may feed normally.

5.24 CASE HISTORY

James was born at 34 weeks gestation by caesarean section, following a period of unsatisfactory intrauterine growth. Following intubation, he breathed unaided for a few hours before developing 'grunting' respirations and sternal recession.

Using the above information, answer the five questions below:

(i) **The baby's respiratory problem is likely to be:**
- **A** Tay-Sach's disease
- **B** pneumonia
- **C** tracheo-oesophageal fistula
- **D** pulmonary surfactant deficiency disease

(ii) **Oxygen concentration should be carefully monitored by:**
- **A** pO_2 levels in the blood
- **B** flowmeter readings
- **C** the degree of cyanosis
- **D** pH levels in the blood

(iii) **Excessive oxygen therapy can cause:**
- **A** intraventricular haemorrhage
- **B** pulmonary stenosis
- **C** retrolental fibroplasia
- **D** achlorhydria

(iv) **In addition to its respiratory problems, the infant may develop convulsions and apnoeic attacks. These are likely to be due to:**
- **A** hypernatraemia
- **B** hypoglycaemia
- **C** Tay-Sach's disease
- **D** proteinuria

(v) **Physiological jaundice will be likely to occur, and should the serum bilirubin level exceed 340 micromols/litre, the following treatment may become necessary:**
- **A** phototherapy
- **B** oral phenobarbitone
- **C** replacement (exchange) transfusion
- **D** electrophoresis

(*answers overleaf*)

5.24

(i) **D**

(ii) **A**

(iii) **C**

It is important for these small babies who need intensive respiratory support to have their blood pO_2 well controlled, so that they will not develop retrolental fibroplasia at a later date, which would mean almost certain blindness.

(iv) **B**

Following intra-uterine growth retardation, this is an important hazard for the baby, and early feeding must be started via a nasogastric tube, or by the intravenous route if necessary.

(v) **C**

In small immature babies, severe physiological jaundice may not respond adequately to phototherapy, and can occasionally require a replacement (exchange) transfusion.

SECTION II
MULTIPLE RESPONSE QUESTIONS Questions 5.25–5.57

Select any number of correct responses between 1–5.

5.25 The newborn baby has:
A a head circumference of 38–40 cm
B an average length at term of 50–54 cm
C an apex beat of over 100 beats per minute
D vernix caseosa
E linea nigra

5.26 Which of the following reflexes are present in the normal neonate at birth:
A sucking
B coughing
C swallowing
D rooting
E bladder control

5.27 Caput succedaneum:
A is a pathological condition
B is oedema caused by cervical pressure on the scalp
C disappears quickly after birth
D occurs only on the head
E crosses suture lines

5.28 Cephalhaematoma:
A is an intracranial haemorrhage
B can cause jaundice
C does not cross suture lines
D may take 6–8 weeks to resolve
E is subperiosteal bleeding of any of the vault bones of the skull

5.29 The condition of the infant at birth may be adjudged satisfactory if:
A the extremities are limp
B facial cyanosis is present
C the apex beat is more than 100 b.p.m.
D gentle stimuli produce a cry
E respiratory movements are established in 30 seconds

(*answers overleaf*)

5.25 **B C D**
The average head circumference is in the range 32–36 cm. Unless the baby is over 4500 g one should be suspicious of a circumference as great as 38–40 cm in case it is an early sign of hydrocephaly.

5.26 **A B C D**

5.27 **B C E**
Caput is not pathological, and may occur on *any* presenting part to which the cervix becomes applied, e.g. swollen external genitalia in a breech.

5.28 **B C D E**
Large or multiple cephalhaematomata can lead to jaundice, especially in immature babies, as a considerable quantity of haemolysed blood has to be absorbed. However, the bleeding is quite definitely under the periosteum, and *not* intracranial.

5.29 **B C D E**
There should be reasonable muscle tone and activity in the infant who responds quickly at birth. However, it is quite normal for there to be facial cyanosis for the first few minutes.

5.30 If a newly delivered baby is pale, limp and shows no sign of respiratory effort, the following could be undertaken by the midwife, while awaiting the arrival of a doctor:

- **A** tracheostomy
- **B** place baby on a resuscitation trolley
- **C** aspirate air passages with a mucus extractor
- **D** ventilate with bag and mask
- **E** endotracheal intubation.

5.31 A baby that is born showing no signs of life after 28 weeks of pregnancy is a:

- **A** spontaneous abortion
- **B** neonatal death
- **C** stillbirth
- **D** perinatal death
- **E** infant death

5.32 An artificially fed baby is more likely to develop the following, than a breast fed baby:

- **A** hypernatraemia
- **B** hypoglycaemia
- **C** anaemia
- **D** jaundice
- **E** infection

5.33 The pre-term infant may be characterised at birth by the presence of:

- **A** vernix caseosa
- **B** milia
- **C** ranula
- **D** lanugo
- **E** red oedematous skin

5.34 Gestational age may be assessed by:

- **A** the firmness of the ear cartilage
- **B** scarf sign
- **C** serum bilirubin
- **D** alignment of heel to opposite ear
- **E** blood glucose estimation

5.35 The immature baby:

- **A** has a small surface area for its body weight
- **B** is prone to respiratory distress syndrome due to a lack of pulmonary surfactant
- **C** may have apnoeic episodes due to an immature respiratory centre
- **D** has a dry wrinkled skin
- **E** is born at less than 37 weeks gestation

(*answers overleaf*)

5.30 **B C D E**
With an infant who has a low Apgar rating, and definite signs of severe hypoxia, endotracheal intubation may well be the most effective way of ventilating the baby, and getting oxygen to the brain. If the midwife does not feel capable of attempting this, she should aspirate the lower pharynx, preferably under direct vision (using a laryngoscope), and then insert an airway, and try bag and mask or mouth-to-mouth/nose resuscitation.

5.31 **C D**
Perinatal mortality includes any baby who is stillborn or dies in the first week of life.

5.32 **A E**
Artificial feeds are fortified with iron, and bottle fed babies are generally overfed rather than underfed! Jaundice affects both bottles and breast fed babies, but there are more opportunities for the introduction of infection with artificial feeding, and even with well-modified cow's milk, overconcentrated feeds can still give the infant an excess of sodium.

5.33 **A D E**
A ranula is a mucus gland retention cyst found in the floor of the mouth.

5.34 **A B D**
Various sets of criteria have been devised to assess gestational age, e.g. Dubovitz score.

5.35 **B C E**
The immature baby tends to have a red, oedematous skin, and *large* surface area for its body weight.

5.36 Hydrocephaly:
- **A** is usually associated with oesophageal atresia
- **B** shows a markedly reduced head circumference
- **C** may often present as a breech in late pregnancy
- **D** can cause cephalo-pelvic disproportion
- **E** causes craniostenosis

5.37 A 'small-for-gestational age' infant:
- **A** has suffered intra-uterine growth retardation
- **B** may be mature or immature
- **C** has a tendency to hypoglycaemia
- **D** usually has a single umbilical artery
- **E** is most common in Social Classes I and II

5.38 Which of the following are *serious* forms of neonatal infection:
- **A** pemphigus neonatorum
- **B** milia
- **C** gonococcal ophthalmia neonatorum
- **D** choanal atresia
- **E** meningitis

5.39 Which of the following congenital abnormalities may be found when examining the head of a newly-delivered infant in the labour ward:
- **A** cleft soft palate
- **B** Pierre-Robin syndrome
- **C** cephalhaematoma
- **D** buphthalmos
- **E** microcephaly

5.40 Jaundice may be caused by:
- **A** septicaemia
- **B** congenital hypothyroidism
- **C** galactosaemia
- **D** rhesus iso-immunisation
- **E** glucose-6-phosphate dehydrogenase deficiency

5.41 Acute abdominal distension in the pre-term infant may indicate:
- **A** necrotising enterocolitis
- **B** meconium ileus
- **C** retrolental fibroplasia
- **D** kernicterus
- **E** inspissated milk curds

(*answers overleaf*)

5.36 **C D**

Hydrocephaly is often associated with some form of spina bifida. The head circumference is increased, and the fontanelles and sutures remain widely open, which is the opposite of craniostenosis, where they fuse prematurely.

5.37 **A B C**

Intra-uterine growth retardation can affect the fetus at any stage of its development. However, where poor placental function inhibits normal growth near to term, the fetus has already made most of its growth, but may lose much of its fat and glycogen stores and thus be classified as 'light-for-gestational age' (dysmature) at birth.

5.38 **A C E**

Choanal atresia is a congenital obstruction of the nasal airway causing respiratory difficulties.
Pemphigus neonatorum is a severe skin infection with bullous skin eruptions. It is usually caused by a virulent strain of staphylococcus, and can easily become epidemic in maternity units.

5.39 **A B D E**

Remember that a cleft soft palate may only be *felt* rather than seen. Buphthalmos is congenital glaucoma, where the affected eye is abnormally large.
Pierre-Robin syndrome is characterised by a very small lower jaw with lax muscles, so that the tongue may fall back and obstruct the air passages. Cephalhaematoma is *not* a congenital anomaly, and is not present at birth.

5.40 **A B C D E**

5.41 **A B E**

Necrotising enterocolitis appears to be more common now that intensive neonatal care is salvaging more very low birth weight babies. Severe infection may be a complicating factor, and perforation of the gut may necessitate surgical resection. The mortality remains high. Inspissated milk curds are usually only troublesome in artificially fed, low birth weight babies, and very occasionally require operative removal of the obstructing curds.

5.42 Twins:
- **A** occur approximately 1 in 80 births
- **B** may be binovular or uniovular
- **C** are usually born by spontaneous vaginal delivery
- **D** are all familial
- **E** have an increased perinatal mortality and morbidity

5.43 Neonatal tetany:
- **A** is treated with intramuscular vitamin K_1
- **B** is usually seen towards the end of the first week of life
- **C** may involve repeated fits
- **D** is diagnosed when the serum calcium is below 1.7 mmol/l (7 mg/100 ml)
- **E** can be associated with a low plasma magnesium.

5.44 The 'light-for-gestational age' infant born near to term:
- **A** is usually hypoglycaemic
- **B** commonly develops pulmonary surfactant deficiency disease
- **C** suffered intrauterine malnutrition
- **D** may have a history of poor placental function tests
- **E** has poor muscle tone, and much vernix

5.45 Rhesus iso-immunisation may occur
- **A** following feto-maternal haemorrhage
- **B** when a rhesus negative woman is pregnant with a rhesus positive fetus
- **C** with ABO incompatibility
- **D** following abortion or antepartum haemorrhage
- **E** due to eclampsia

5.46 Kernicterus is characterised by:
- **A** convulsions
- **B** head retraction
- **C** talipes
- **D** rolling of the eyes
- **E** mental retardation

5.47 The baby born to a diabetic mother:
- **A** is often born by caesarean section
- **B** always inherits diabetes mellitus
- **C** is predisposed to meconium ileus
- **D** is usually delivered 1–2 weeks before term
- **E** is prone to respiratory problems

(*answers overleaf*)

5.42 **A B E**

Only binovular twins are familial, and due to the high incidence of malpresentation, instrumental or even operative delivery is common.

5.43 **B C D E**

Neonatal tetany usually occurs in artificially fed babies, although it has become less common now that cow's milk preparations are better modified, and have a reduced phosphorus content, as a high phosphate load probably interferes with the absorption of calcium. The initial treatment is i.v. calcium gluconate 10 per cent given *slowly*, and i.m. magnesium sulphate, if hypomagnesaemia is also a problem.

5.44 **A C D**

Excessive vernix, hypotonia, and a deficiency of surfactant are associated with significant prematurity.

5.45 **A B D**

ABO incompatibility, unlike rhesus iso-immunisation, can occur in a first pregnancy, as it is due to incompatibility between the maternal and fetal ABO group with the production of specific ABO antibodies. The prediction of severity is less easy than with rhesus disease, but haemolysis will occur, and the baby may be jaundiced and require phototherapy, or even exchange transfusion.

5.46 **A B D E**

These severe sequelae are caused by the basal ganglia absorbing high levels of toxic, fat-soluble, unconjugated bilirubin.

5.47 **A D E**

Only a small proportion of babies born to diabetics will develop diabetes mellitus.
Caesarean section is still a common method of delivery for the diabetic mother, but improvement in the control of maternal diabetes in pregnancy is leading to an increasing number of moderately-sized infants being delivered by the vaginal route.
When diabetes is well controlled throughout the pregnancy, the fetal outcome is generally good. However, where control is poor babies may still be born overweight or growth-retarded and have respiratory problems.

5.48 An infant with Down's syndrome (Trisomy 21) often has:
- **A** a flat occiput
- **B** a single palmar crease
- **C** a bulging anterior fontanelle
- **D** 46 chromosomes
- **E** hypotonicity

5.49 The following congenital conditions are sex-linked:
- **A** Down's syndrome
- **B** haemophilia
- **C** Duchenne muscular dystrophy
- **D** phenylketonuria
- **E** galactosaemia

5.50 Ophthalmia neonatorum:
- **A** is any inflammation occurring in the infant's eyes within 14 days of birth
- **B** is a purulent discharge from the infant's eyes within 21 days of birth
- **C** must be reported to the doctor
- **D** must be notified by the dotor to the District Health Authority
- **E** can be caused by untreated syphilis in the mother

5.51 In severe cases of pulmonary surfactant deficiency disease, respiration may be supported by:
- **A** cardiac monitor
- **B** electro-cardiograph
- **C** continuous positive airways pressure(CPAP)
- **D** intermittent positive pressure ventilation
- **E** Spitz-Holter valve

5.52 The very immature infant has difficulty maintaining his body temperature because he has:
- **A** low glycogen stores in his liver and muscles
- **B** a large surface area to body weight ratio
- **C** only small amounts of brown fat
- **D** poor subcutaneous fat insulation
- **E** an immature respiratory centre

5.53 Which of the following are inherited through a *dominant* gene, i.e. only one abnormal gene will produce the defect:
- **A** Marfan's syndrome
- **B** phenylketonuria
- **C** achondroplasia
- **D** galactosaemia
- **E** hypospadias

(*answers overleaf*)

5.48 **A B E**
Due to the extra chromosome on the 21 pair of autosomes, these infants have *47* chromosomes.

5.49 **B C**
Examples of sex-linked diseases are haemophilia and the severe (Duchenne) form of muscular dystrophy. Both are carried by the female, who is unaffected, and generally transmitted to half her male children. Phenylketonuria and galactosaemia are inherited as autosomal recessive characteristics, both parents being heterozygous carriers, and they have a 1:4 risk of producing an affected child.

5.50 **B C D**
Gonococcal ophthalmia neonatorum can cause blindness, and is a notifiable disease, so that by law, the doctor in charge of the case must inform the District Health Authority.

5.51 **C D**
A cardio-rater and ECG may well be used with an infant needing artificial ventilation or C.P.A.P., but they do not give respiratory support. In hydrocephaly a Spitz-Holter valve is used to by-pass a blockage in the ventricular canal system of the brain, so that a build up of cerebro-spinal fluid does not cause irreversible brain damage.

5.52 **A B C D**
The immature respiratory centre is not concerned in the maintenance of body temperature!

5.53 **A C**
In these diseases, only one gene will produce the disease, which is why it is called *dominant* genetic inheritance.

5.54 Congenital abnormality in the infant is more commonly seen when:

A a single umbilical artery is present
B the mother is a diabetic
C one umbilical vein is present
D the mother is aged 40 years or over
E the placenta is bipartite

5.55 The following are causes of *persistent* neonatal jaundice:

A artificial milk feeding
B biliary atresia
C hypothyroidism
D coryza
E vitamin D deficiency

(*answers overleaf*)

5.54 **A B D**
A single umbilical artery is often associated with another congenital anomaly (e.g. renal agenesis).
The incidence of congenital abnormality in babies born to diabetics is approximately 4 per cent, which is roughly double the figure for non-diabetics, and women over 40 have a steadily increasing incidence of Trisomy 21 (Down's syndrome).

5.55 **B C**
With congenital hypothyroidism (cretinism), the jaundice is usually mild, but with biliary atresia, where the bile ducts are congenitally absent, the jaundice presents late, and increases in severity. Only about 10 per cent are operable, and the remainder perish at 18 months-2 years, although liver transplant may offer a solution in the future.

5.56 CASE HISTORY

A male infant weighing 4000 g arrives in the Special Care Baby Unit following a difficult breech delivery at 39 weeks gestation. Apgar scores at 1 and 5 minutes were 1 and 3 respectively, following immediate endotracheal intubation and ventilation. Using the above information, answer the following three questions. For questions (i) and (ii) select any number of correct responses between 1–5.

(i) This baby is likely to suffer from which of the following:

A meconium aspiration into the lungs
B pulmonary surfactant deficiency disease
C excessive moulding
D hypoglycaemia
E intracranial haemorrhage

(ii) This baby should be examined with particular care, for the following birth injuries, which characteristically are associated with difficult breech delivery:

A rupture of the adrenal glands
B fracture of the humerus
C hypoxic brain damage
D pneumothorax
E oedematous scrotum

(iii) Indicate whether the following statements are 'true' or 'false':

A The optimum weight for the baby, if delivered as a breech, is between 2500–3000 g
B The Burns-Marshall manoeuvre is a technique used to deliver extended arms
C Severe intracranial haemorrhage following breech delivery, is often caused by a tentorial tear
D The Mauriceau-Smellie-Veit manoeuvre is used to flex the after-coming head to facilitate delivery
E The incidence of breech presentation in labour is between 2–3 per cent

(*answers overleaf*)

5.56

(i) **A E**

(ii) **A B C E**
Evidence of hypoxic brain damage may not be obvious initially, and these babies should be carefully followed up during the first years of life. Rupture of abdominal organs such as the liver, spleen, kidneys or adrenals can occur if the baby is grasped round the *abdomen* (instead of the pelvis) during a difficult breech delivery. An extended arm can lie awkwardly behind the head, and may be fractured during attempts to release it. The external genitalia in both male and female babies can be severely bruised and oedematous following repeated vaginal examinations and the constricting action of the cervix during labour.

(iii) **A True**
The mortality and morbidity rates rise significantly for babies lighter or heavier than this range, when they are vaginal breech deliveries

B False
The Burns-Marshall manoeuvre is used to deliver the well flexed after-coming head of a breech. Løvset's manoeuvre is used to deliver extended arms.

C True

D True

E True

True
Moulding does not take place, as the after-coming head is so rapidly compressed to enter the pelvis during the second stage of labour, and unless good control of the head is maintained throughout delivery, rapid decompression may occur as the head escapes from the birth canal, and it is this that can cause intracranial haemorrhage.

5.57 *Figure* 12

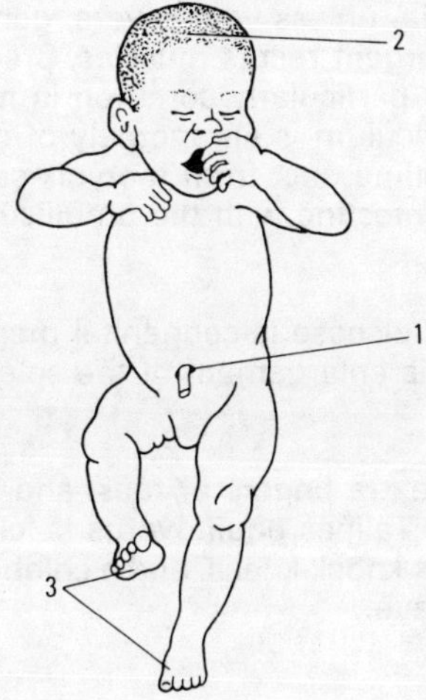

This question relates to the above diagram.
Identify the congenital abnormalities which may be associated with each region numbered 1–3.

1
- **A** hydrocele
- **B** umbilical hernia
- **C** Meckel's diverticulum
- **D** divergent rectus abdominis muscles
- **E** hypospadias

2.
- **A** Hirschsprung's disease
- **B** polydactyly
- **C** hydrocephaly
- **D** splenomegaly
- **E** craniostenosis

3.
- **A** polydactyly
- **B** talipes equinovarus
- **C** syndactyly
- **D** genu valgum
- **E** coloboma

(*answers overleaf*)

5.57

1 **B C D**

Umbilical hernia, unless very severe, generally needs no treatment. Divergent rectus muscles, predispose to the above, and are particularly common in negro children. Meckel's diverticulum is an anomaly of development, where part of the vitelline duct from the yolk sac persists, and may link the small intestine with the umbilicus.

2 **C E**

Hirschsprung's disease is congenital megacolon, and splenomegaly is enlargement of the spleen.

3 **A B C**

Polydactyly is extra fingers or toes, and syndactyly is webbed digits. Talipes equinovarus is 'club foot'. Genu valgum is knock-knees, and a coloboma is a defect of the iris of the eye.

SECTION III
TRUE OR FALSE? Questions 5.58–5.72

Indicate whether you think the statements listed below are true or false.

5.58 Where the mother contracts rubella in early pregnancy, the infant can be born many months later with the active form of the disease.

5.59 Infection of the fetus with cytomegalovirus can cause severe mental subnormality and deafness in the child.

5.60 Necrotising enterocolitis is associated with extreme prematurity, and umbilical vein or artery catheterisation.

5.61 Blood volume in the normal, mature neonate can be calculated at approximately 200 ml per kilogram body weight.

5.62 The ductus arteriosus usually closes within a few hours of birth, but may remain patent, particularly if the infant is hypoxic and difficult to resuscitate.

5.63 An infant who dies within the first year of life is classified as an infant death.

5.64 Cephalhaematoma is best treated by aspiration.

5.65 The pallor associated with severe birth asphyxia is caused by a reduction in the peripheral circulation.

5.66 By the end of the first week of life the normal mature baby requires approximately 100 ml of milk feed per kilo per day.

5.67 Sudden unexpected infant deaths are more common in artificially-fed babies than in those that are fully breast-fed.

5.68 Newborn babies produce copious tears when they cry.

(*answers overleaf*)

5.58 **True**
In addition, the infant may demonstrate any of the classical congenital defects associated with this disease, e.g. microcephaly, deafness, cataract, heart defects.

5.59 **True**
Cytomegalovirus (CMV) is excreted in 1–3 per cent of all neonates. Most of them are perfectly normal, but a few may be damaged or even stillborn. The virus involves the central nervous system particularly, and the infant may present with jaundice, respiratory problems, fits, and mental retardation.

5.60 **True**

5.61 **False**
Blood volume can be calculated at approximately 85 ml/kg body weight, i.e. an infant weighing 3 kg has a blood volume of about 255 ml.

5.62 **True**

5.63 **True**
This will include all those who are also classified as neonatal and 'first week' deaths.

5.64 **False**
Cephalhaematoma will resolve spontaneously, and should definitely *not* be aspirated, as this may introduce infection. However it may persist for 6–8 weeks, and the parents must receive an explicit explanation and reassurance.

5.65 **True**
When oxygen deprivation in the fetus is prolonged, the peripheral circulation is markedly reduced so conserving what oxygen there is for the vital centres.

5.66 **False**
150 ml per kilo per day is the commonly accepted formula once feeding is fully established.

5.67 **True**
Although a small number of 'cot deaths' do occur in breast-fed infants.

5.68 **False**
Newborn infants do not produce copious tears initially, which is one reason why they may be prone to 'sticky eyes'.

5.69 Vernix caseosa protects the skin from maceration during intra-uterine life.

5.70 The newborn baby has an enlarged liver at birth.

5.71 The infant who suffers from intra-uterine malnutrition in the last few weeks of pregnancy is termed 'light-for-gestational age' when born near to term.

5.72 If the cord blood haemoglobin level is below 10 g/dl and the unconjugated serum bilirubin is above 170 micromol/litre, immediate replacement (exchange) transfusion would be indicated.

5.73 Vaginal bleeding in the neonate is usually due to a severe vaginal 'thrush' infection (candidiasis).

(*answers overleaf*)

5.69 **True**
Following intra-uterine death the fetal tissues undergo softening and degeneration with fluid accumulating under the epidermis, and this is termed maceration.

5.70 **True**
It is normal for the neonate to have a slightly enlarged liver, palpable 2–4 cm below the right costal margin.

5.71 **True**

5.72 **True**
In the normal newborn baby the haemoglobin would be 16–20 g/dl, so a level of 10 g/dl would indicate severe anaemia, and allied with a high serum bilirubin in the *cord* blood, an exchange transfusion would seem essential.

5.73 **False**
Scanty vaginal bleeding seen in the first week of life is usually 'pseudomenstruation' caused by the fall in circulating maternal steroids (e.g. oestrogens) following birth.

SECTION IV
MATCHING ITEMS Questions 5.74–5.79

Match the items in Group 1 with the most appropriate item in Group 2. (Each item in Group 2 can only be used *once*.)

5.74 Match the items in Group 1 with the most appropriate item in Group 2.

Group 1		*Group 2*
(i) dry gangrene	**A**	haemophilia
(ii) draught reflex	**B**	prematurity
(iii) lanugo	**C**	umbilical cord stump
(iv) hyperbilirubinaemia	**D**	haemolytic disease
	E	breast feeding

5.75 Match the items in Group 1 with the most appropriate item in Group 2.

Group 1		*Group 2*
(i) hard, green stool	**A**	imperforate anus
(ii) loose, offensive green stool	**B**	Hirschsprung's disease
(iii) absence of stools	**C**	gastro-enteritis
(iv) megacolon	**D**	pilonidal sinus
	E	underfed baby

5.76 Match the items in Group 1 with the most appropriate item in Group 2.

Group 1		*Group 2*
(i) soft, bright yellow stool	**A**	artifically fed baby
(ii) firm, pale yellow stool	**B**	haemorrhagic disease
(iii) brownish, yellow stool	**C**	breast fed baby
(iv) reddish brown stool	**D**	gastro-enteritis
	E	changing stool

5.77 Match the items in Group 1 with the most appropriate item in Group 2.

Group 1		*Group 2*
(i) artificial feeding	**A**	Spalding's sign
(ii) extreme prematurity	**B**	lack of pulmonary surfactant
(iii) breech delivery	**C**	intraventricular haemorrhage
(iv) respiratory distress syndrome	**D**	hypernatraemia
	E	tentorial tear

(*answers overleaf*)

5.74

(i) **C**
(ii) **E**
(iii) **B**
(iv) **D**

5.75

(i) **E**
(ii) **C**
(iii) **A**
(iv) **B**

5.76

(i) **C**
(ii) **A**
(iii) **E**
(iv) **B**

5.77

(i) **D**
(ii) **C**
(iii) **E**
(iv) **B**

5.78 Match the items in Group 1 with the most appropriate item in Group 2.

Group 1		*Group 2*
(i) Coomb's test	**A**	'light-for-gestational age' infants
(ii) Guthrie test	**B**	rhesus iso-immunisation
(iii) Hutchinson's teeth	**C**	congenital syphilis
(iv) hypoglycaemia	**D**	phenylketonuria
	E	ophthalmia neonatorum

5.79 Match the items in Group 1 with the most appropriate item in Group 2.

Group 1		*Group 2*
(i) Barlow's test	**A**	breast feeding
(ii) BCG vaccination	**B**	congenital dislocation of the hip
(iii) lactalbumin	**C**	haemolytic disease
(iv) vitamin K_1	**D**	haemorrhagic disease
	E	pulmonary tuberculosis

(*answers overleaf*)

5.78

(i) **B**
(ii) **D**
(iii) **C**
(iv) **A**

5.79

(i) **B**
(ii) **E**
(iii) **A**
(iv) **D**

SECTION V
ASSERTION/REASON QUESTIONS 5.80–5.87

Read carefully the five possible answers listed below marked **A, B, C, D** and **E**. Select which is appropriate for the assertions and reasons which follow.

A Assertion true; reason is a true statement, and is the correct reason.
B Assertion and reason both true, but reason is *not* the correct reason.
C Assertion is true, but reason is a false statement.
D Assertion is false, but the reason is a true statement.
E Assertion and reason are both false.

5.80 The mature infant at birth has a high haemoglobin level in the range of 10–12 g/dl
because
the placenta is a more efficient organ of respiration for the fetus, than are the lungs of the baby.

5.81 Pre-term infants should have a daily intake of vitamin D 800 units
because
they have an increased tendency to develop rickets.

5.82 At birth the foreskin should never be retracted forcibly
because
it is firmly adherent to the glans penis, and will gradually separate and retract by the time the boy is about 3 years old.

5.83 Physiological jaundice most commonly occurs on the sixth to seventh day of life
because
The immature liver produces inadequate glucuronyl transferase.

5.84 The pre-term infant has particular difficulty in maintaining his body temperature
because
he is deficient in subcutaneous fat for insulation and metabolism.

5.85 Umbilical cord stump infections may lead to septicaemia
because
the ductus venosus communicates directly with the hypogastric arteries.

(*answers overleaf*)

5.80 **E**

The mature neonate has a high haemoglobin level (16–20 g/dl) due to the fact that there are about 1 million extra red cells needed during intrauterine life, and these are only gradually reduced over the first few weeks of extrauterine life. The reason for these extra red cells is that the placenta is a *less* efficient organ of respiration than the mature lungs.

5.81 **A**

Most modified cow's milk preparations contain a suitable supplement of vitamin D.

5.82 **A**

5.83 **D**

Physiological jaundice is most commonly seen from the third or fourth day of life. There is an additional load on the liver because of the excess red cells being broken down in the first few days of life. Glucuronyl transferase is the liver enzyme which converts fat-soluble bilirubin to water-soluble, a process often called conjugation.

5.84 **A**

The pre-term infant is prone to hypothermia not only because he lacks the insulation of a layer of subcutaneous fat, but also because he has reduced brown fat stores, a large surface area to weight ratio, and is unable to shiver when he becomes chilled.

5.85 **C**

The ductus venosus communicates directly with the inferior vena cava, while the hypogastric arteries are continuous with the umbilical arteries.

5.86 **A positive Coomb's test on the cord blood usually indicates haemolytic disease**
because
a positive Coomb's test demonstrates the presence of rhesus or ABO antibodies in the fetal circulation, and these antibodies haemolyse red blood cells.

5.87 **Haemorrhagic disease of the newborn is now comparatively uncommon**
because
most rhesus negative women are treated prophylactically with Anti-D immunoglobulin.

(*answers overleaf*)

5.86 **C**
A positive Coomb's test demonstrates the presence of maternal Rhesus antibodies in the fetal/neonatal circulation, and in a rhesus positive fetus or baby these antibodies cause haemolysis.

5.87 **B**

SECTION VI
COMPLETION ITEMS Questions 5.88–5.95

Supply the missing word (s) in the following statements:

5.88 **All mothers should be encouraged to talk to and handle their babies early on, as this promotes good____________.**

5.89 **Necrosis of the scalp with subsequent hair loss can be a complication following a traumatic delivery by____________.**

5.90 **In the breast fed baby, a small melaena stool may occasionally be due to____________rather than haemorrhagic disease.**

5.91 **Long-term ventilation via an endotracheal tube in extremely immature infants may eventually lead to a____________.**

5.92 **Oesophageal atresia is frequently associated with a____________.**

5.93 **Besides encouraging good 'bonding', early____________ also promotes rapid colonisation of the gut with non-pathogenic organisms from the mother.**

5.94 **Pulmonary haemorrhage may be a terminal event, and is most commonly seen in____________babies.**

(*answers overleaf*)

5.88 Emotional 'bonding' (attachment)

5.89 Vacuum (Ventouse) extraction

5.90 Cracked nipples in the mother

5.91 Tracheal stenosis

5.92 Tracheo-oesophageal fistula

5.93 Breast feeding

5.94 Low birth weight/'light-for-gestational age'
Pulmonary haemorrhage is generally fatal, and often follows respiratory difficulties, severe infections or hypothermia in these already disadvantaged babies.

CASE HISTORY.

5.95 **Susan is 24-hours-old. At birth she weighed 2200 g following a precipitate delivery at 36 weeks gestation. She now has large bilateral cephalhaematomata situated over the parietal bones. (A cephaelhaematoma is a collection of blood under the____________and can occur over other skull bones i.e. the____________and____________ bones.)**

As Susan was born prematurely, the cephalhaematomata, are likely to cause significant____________, which may need to be treated with____________. or if very severe, by____________transfusion.

Soon after birth Susan was given an i.m. injection of____________ to prevent____________disease of the newborn, which could follow a very rapid delivery.

This substance is necessary for the production of____________ in the liver, which is an essential constituent for blood coagulation.

Following precipitate delivery, intracranial haemorrhage can occur, and Susan is observed closely for signs such as____________ any of which could indicate an intracranial bleed.
Susan's parents are encouraged to spend time with her, and to share in her care, as this helps to promote good____________

(*answers overleaf*)

5.95 a periosteum
b occiput and frontal bones
c Jaundice— All infants, and especially the premature, have difficulty in producing enough liver enzyme (gluceronyl transferase) to convert the major red cell breakdown product, bilirubin, from a toxic fat soluble compound to a water soluble substance which can be excreted via the urine and faeces.
An additional influx of red cell breakdown products from a cephalhaematoma may overload the system disastrously and can cause very high levels of unconjugated bilirubin with the risk of kernicterus if untreated.

d Phototherapy
e Exchange (replacement) transfusion
f Vitamin K_1 (Konakion) 0.5–1.0 mg

g Haemorrhagic (disease of the newborn)
h Prothrombin
In haemorrhagic disease the baby suddenly begins to bleed, usually 2–4 days after birth and most commonly from the alimentary tract, but can be from any site. It is most frequently seen in pre-term, breastfed babies who have a low prothrombin level.

i twitching, irritability or convulsions
lack of muscle tone
vomiting
apnoeic attacks
shrill cry
tense fontanelle
pallor
hypothermia

j Emotional bonding

NEONATAL PAEDIATRICS

The following questions are taken from recent examination papers set by the English National Board.

1. Essay questions

How would you anticipate and recognise an infant with severe birth asphyxia? Describe in detail how the midwife would resuscitate such a baby. (1983)

What neonatal problems and complications may arise following planned early transfer? How would these be dealt with by the midwife? (1983)

What are the basic needs of a healthy full-term infant? Illustrate how these needs may be met during the neonatal period. (1983)

Which babies are at particular risk of cerebral trauma? What measures can be taken to help prevent injury? Give the signs of cerebral trauma and describe the full nursing care. (1983)

Describe the role of the midwife in the care of a baby during the neonatal period. What observations and records should she make? (1983)

How may the midwife help to prevent and recognise infection in the baby during the first 28 days of life? (1983)

A baby is born at 32 weeks gestation weighing 1.7 kg. Describe the care that this preterm baby may require, highlighting the problems which may arise. (1983)

What may make the midwife or the mother suspect that a full term baby is not progressing normally in the first week of life? How should this be investigated? (1983)

List the causes of jaundice in the newborn. Describe the management of an infant who develops jaundice within the first 24 hours of life. (1984)

What are the signs of severe hypothermia in the neonate? Describe the management of a baby with this condition. How may hypothermia be prevented? (1984)

What would make a midwife suspect that a baby has an oesphageal atresia?
What are the dangers of this condition? (1984)

List the possible causes of vomiting during the neonatal period. What observations should the midwife make which, together with the information she receives from the mother, assist in making a diagnosis? (1984)

Describe the normal physiological changes which occur in the fetus during labour and the birth process, which assist the baby to adapt to its new environment. How would you monitor these changes? (1984)

What is the composition of human breast milk?
How should cow's milk be modified to make it suitable for the neonate?
What are the advantages to the baby of breast feeding? (1984)

Explain how congenital abnormalities may be diagnosed during the first 10 days of life.
Describe the midwife's responsibilities in this connection. (1984)

How is the baby's condition assessed at birth?
Describe in detail the action the midwife should take when the baby fails to breathe after delivery. (1984)

What is immunity? How may a baby acquire immunity
a. in the neonatal period?
b. during childhood? (1985)

Describe the admission of a baby to the postnatal ward. What are the midwife's responsibilities, and how might she provide optimum care within the first 48 hours? (1985)

Following a difficult vaginal delivery at 40 weeks gestation a male infant weighing 3500 g is admitted to the Special Care Baby Unit. State the probable reasons for admission and describe the care that may be necessary for the baby during the first week of life. (1985)

2. **Write briefly on each of the following subjects:**
Stools of the infant in the first week of life (1983)
Assessing the maturity of a pre-term infant (1983)
Diagnosis of Down's Syndrome (1983)
Apgar score (1983)
Oesophageal atresia (1983)
Characteristics of the pre-term infant (1983)
Prevention of neonatal hypothermia (1983)
Recognition of respiratory distress syndrome (1983)
Congenital dislocation of the hips (1983)
Sore buttocks (1983)
Physiological jaundice (1983)
Babies at risk of developing hypoglycaemia (1983)
Follow up of the normal baby from the tenth day of life (1983)
Necrotising enterocolitis (1983)
Neonatal thrush (1983)
Hazards to the baby of being cared for in an incubator (1983)

Immediate care of the neonate at birth (1984)
Effects on the neonate of severe fetal hypoxia in labour (1984)
The skin of the neonate (1984)
Causes of vomiting in the first week of life (1984)
Administration of drugs to the neonate (1984)
Prevention of cross infection in a Special Care Baby Unit (1984)
Significance of the neonatal neurological reflexes (1984)
Ophthalmia neonatorum (1984)
Phototherapy (1984)
Neonatal hypoglycaemia (1984)
Care of the umbilical cord (1984)
Melaena (1984)
Recognition at birth of a growth retarded baby (1984)
Interpretation of a baby's cry (1984)
Reasons why babies are reluctant to feed (1984)
Role of Special Baby Care Units (1984)
ABO incompatibility (1985)
Recognition of cerebral irritation (1985)
Heat regulation in the newborn (1985)
Causes of cyanosis in the first week of life (1985)

6. Community health

At the present time the Government is proposing radical changes in social benefits, which if implemented after the publication of this edition, could invalidate certain questions and answers.

SECTION I
SINGLE RESPONSE MULTIPLE CHOICE QUESTIONS Questions 6.1–6.44

Select a *single* correct response to each of the following questions:

6.1 The stillbirth rate is the number of infants who are born dead after 28 weeks of pregnancy per:
A 1000 total births
B 1000 live births
C 100 000 total births
D 10 000 live and still births

6.2 The most important reason for the dramatic reduction in maternal mortality between 1935–1960 was:
A improved nutrition and housing
B better obstetric practice
C the National Health Service
D improved blood transfusion and antibiotic therapy

6.3 The neonatal death rate per 1000 live births is defined as:
A deaths occurring in the first month of life
B deaths occurring in the first week of life
C deaths occurring in the first year of life
D deaths ocurring in the first 24 hours of life

6.4 Maternal mortality is the number of maternal deaths which occur per 1000 total births, as a direct result of:
A abortion, delivery and the puerperium
B pregnancy, childbirth and the puerperium
C delivery and the postnatal period
D abortion and haemorrhage

(*answers overleaf*)

6.1 **A**
(Stillbirth rate (19______)__________________per 1000 total births.)*

6.2 **D**
An efficient blood transfusion service, and the use of chemotherapy and antibiotics, produced the most dramatic fall in maternal mortality, as it reduced the deaths due to puerperal sepsis and haemorrhage. The other factors also played a lesser, but continuing role in reducing maternal deaths.

6.3 **A**
(Neonatal mortality (19______)__________________per 1000 live births.)*

6.4 **B**
(Maternal mortality (19______)__________________per 1000 total births.)*

*Statistics alter frequently, so fill in the most recent figure in the space provided, as an aid to your revision.

6.5 **The perinatal death rate is composed of stillbirths and______ calculated per 1000 total births.**
- **A** first day deaths
- **B** first week deaths
- **C** neonatal deaths
- **D** infant deaths

6.6 **Infant mortality refers to babies who die:**
- **A** as unexpected 'cot deaths'
- **B** as a result of infection
- **C** in the first month of life
- **D** in the first year of life

6.7 **The Abortion Act was made law in:**
- **A** 1969
- **B** 1968
- **C** 1967
- **D** 1966

6.8 **'Triple vaccine' provides immunisation against:**
- **A** diphtheria, tetanus and polio
- **B** diphtheria, tetanus and pertussis
- **C** Whooping cough, tetanus and measles
- **D** polio, diphtheria and measles

6.9 **What immunisation should be offered to girls aged 10–13 years?**
- **A** smallpox
- **B** measles
- **C** rubella
- **D** tetanus

6.10 **Measles vaccine is usually given at approximately:**
- **A** 3 months
- **B** 6 months
- **C** 15 months
- **D** 5 years

6.11 **Priority for day nursery places is given to:**
- **A** working mothers
- **B** grande multiparae
- **C** primigravidae
- **D** one parent families

(*answers overleaf*)

6.5 **B**
(Perinatal mortality (19_____)__________________per 1000 total births)*

6.6 **D**
(Infant mortality (19_____)__________________per 1000 live births)*

6.7 **C**

6.8 **B**

6.9 **C**

6.10 **C**

6.11 **D**

*Statistics alter frequently, so fill in the most recent figure in the space provided, as an aid to your revision.

6.12 **What is the alternative day care provision for children who cannot be accommodated in day nurseries due to lack of available places?**
A children's homes
B residential nurseries
C play groups
D child minders

6.13 **The most common sexually transmitted disease in women, in this country is:**
A candidiasis
B gonorrhoea
C yaws
D syphilis

6.14 **A chancre is the most prominent diagnostic sign of:**
A non-specific urethritis
B gonorrhoea
C trichomonas vaginalis infection
D primary syphilis

6.15 **A generalised rash is a prominent sign of which phase of syphilis:**
A primary
B secondary
C tertiary
D neurosyphilis

6.16 **The most usual treatment for syphilis is large doses of:**
A sulphonamides
B gentamicin
C paracetamol
D penicillin

6.17 **The organism most frequently causing vaginal infections is:**
A gonococcus
B candida albicans
C treponema pallidum
D clostridium welchii

6.18 **A greenish, slightly frothy vaginal discharge is frequently a sign of infection due to:**
A bacillus proteus
B candida albicans
C trichomonas vaginalis
D chlamydia

(*answers overleaf*)

6.12 **D**

Play groups are not an equal alternative to a day nursery, as they may only function for a few hours each day, which is of little use to a full-time working mother.

6.13 **A**

Most, but not all candidiasis (thrush) is sexually transmitted, and it is a very common complaint.

6.14 **D**

A chancre is a painless ulcer that most commonly occurs on the genitalia. Because it heals quickly, treatment may not be sought, and the early diagnosis of syphilis may be missed.

6.15 **B**

6.16 **D**

The treatment of choice is still large doses of i.m. procaine penicillin for 10–15 days.

6.17 **B**

6.18 **C**

Trichomonas vaginalis is a motile, flagellate protozoan, which causes an intensely irritant vaginal infection.

6.19 The effective drug for destroying *Trichomonas vaginalis* is:
A metronidazole
B methotrexate
C tobramycin
D tetracycline

6.20 Which of the following is a notifiable disease?
A ophthalmia neonatorum
B puerperal sepsis
C puerperal pyrexia
D gas gangrene

6.21 The most *common* causative organism of ophthalmia neonatorum is:
A haemolytic streptococcus
B staphylococcus aureus
C gonococcus
D candida albicans

6.22 Which controlled drugs may a community midwife legally possess?
A morphine and Omnopon
B Fortral and Narphen
C pethidine and Pethilorfan
D methadone and Fortral

6.23 From whom does a community midwife obtain her controlled drug supply orders?
A divisional midwifery officer
B supervisor of midwives
C senior nursing officer
D superintendent midwife

6.24 The local supervising authority is:
A local government
B local midwifery administration of the National Board.
C the corporate management board
D Community Health Council

6.25 At a local level, the designated officer of the local supervising authority is known as the:
A superintendent midwife
B divisional midwifery officer
C senior nursing officer
D supervisor of midwives

(*answers overleaf*)

6.19 **A**
Metronidazole (Flagyl) 200 mg t.d.s. for 7–10 days, given in tablet form. It may also be necessary to treat the sexual partner who may be acting as a symptomless reservoir of infection.

6.20 **A**
This means that the doctor in charge of the case must notify the District Health Authority.

6.21 **B**
The gonococcus is the most damaging organism to infect the eyes, but particularly in maternity units, the *staphylococcus aureus* is a much commoner organism to cause eye infections. Chlamydial eye infections have also become more common.

6.22 **C**
A community midwife may also possess Fortral but it is *not* a controlled drug at the present time, although there is now evidence that this drug is capable of leading to addiction, and there are now initiatives being taken to include it in controlled drug legislation.

6.23 **B**

6.24 **B**
The National Boards delegate statutory supervision of midwifery practice to local supervisors of midwives through the NHS administration, e.g. in England it is the Regional Health Authority.

6.25 **D**
In England, the National Board and the Regional Health Authority approve a number of supervisors of midwives in each health district, who are then chiefly responsible for the local supervision of midwifery practice in their health district.

6.26 The National Boards have the statutory authority to:
A approve and inspect training schools
B remove a midwife's name from the register
C maintain a live register of midwives
D collect annual 'Notifications of Intention to Practice'

6.27 Which of the following is *not* a function of the local supervising authority?
A issue drug supply orders to midwives
B general supervision of all midwives
C conduct penal sessions
D ensure midwives attend refresher courses every five years

6.28 Who normally registers the birth?
A the hospital administrator
B the general practitioner
C the midwife
D the parents

6.29 All births should be registered by the parents within:
A 48 hours of the birth
B 4 weeks of the birth
C 6 weeks of the birth
D 10 weeks of the birth

6.30 Birth notification should be within:
A 24 hours of birth
B 30 hours of birth
C 36 hours of birth
D 48 hours of birth

6.31 Births should be notified by the midwife to:
A District Health Authority
B district management board
C district nursing officer
D district community physician

6.32 A fit woman aged 24 years wishes to have a home confinement. Her doctor may agree if:
A she has had one previous normal delivery
B she has had four previous normal deliveries
C her height is 150 cm
D this is her first pregnancy

(*answers overleaf*)

6.26 **A**
The maintainance of a live register of midwives, and the removal of a midwife's name from that register following disciplinary proceedings is a statutory responsibility of the UK Central Council, while the collection of annual notifications of intention to practise falls to local supervisors of midwives.

6.27 **C**
This is a *central* function of the statutory bodies although the local supervisor of midwives may make *initial* investigations if there is a complaint about a midwife in her health district. The National Boards may initiate action through their Investigating committees, but the UKCC undertakes the formal disciplinary hearings.

6.28 **D**
However, any person present at the birth can register the child in default of the parents.

6.29 **C**

6.30 **C**

6.31 **A**
In law any person present at the birth can notify it to the District Health Authority, but traditionally the midwife always does so.

6.32 **A**

6.33 The Home Help Service is administered by:
A Citizen's Advice Bureau
B Social Services Department
C National Health Service
D primary health care team

6.34 Which of the following is *not* provided by the social services department of the local authority?
A fostering
B day nurseries
C nursery schools
D child minding

6.35 Social work services are provided by:
A National Health Service
B Community Health Service
C Environmental Health Service
D local government

6.36 The National Health Service became functional in:
A 1938
B 1942
C 1948
D 1952

6.37 The National Health Service was first reorganised in:
A 1970
B 1972
C 1973
D 1974

6.38 The single lump sum payment, made to pregnant women, and designed to help with the expenses of a layette, is known as:
A maternity allowance
B maternity grant
C maternity benefit
D family income supplement

6.39 The Maternity Allowance provides:
A supplementary benefits if the family income is low
B tax relief for the new baby
C 18 weekly payments
D one pint of free milk daily

(*answers overleaf*)

6.33 **B**

6.34 **C**
Nursery schools are provided by the Education Department of the local authority.

6.35 **D**
Every local authority (local government) has a Social Services Department which is staffed by social workers.

6.36 **C**

6.37 **D**

6.38 **B***

6.39 **C***
The maternity allowance is paid for a total of 18 weeks, usually 11 weeks before the birth and seven weeks afterwards. Women who have recently been in full time employment are usually eligible.

*The amount payable for these maternity benefits changes frequently, so find out the current figure and fill it in below.
1. Maternity grant £ ____________________ (single payment)
2. Maternity allowance £ ____________________ (basic weekly rate)

6.40 Who is entitled to one pint of free milk a day in pregnancy?

A women claiming the maternity allowance
B women claiming supplementary benefits
C women suffering from anaemia
D grande multiparae

6.41 The second reorganisation of the National Health Service became effective in 1982. One major change was the abolition of:

A district administrators
B Citizen's Advice Bureaux
C Area Health Authorities
D Regional Health Authorities

6.42 Which of these organisations has been described as a 'watchdog' for the NHS consumer?

A health care planning team
B district management team
C community health council
D primary health care team

6.43 General practitioners, community nurses, midwives and health visitors, constitute the basis of:

A primary health care team
B community health council
C health care planning team
D local supervising authority

6.44 The Environmental Health Services are administered by:

A District Health Authority
B local authority
C district community physician
D district management team

(*answers overleaf*)

6.40 **B**
(i.e. women in low income groups)

6.41 **C**

6.42 **C**

6.43 **A**

6.44 **B**
Another department of the local authority that safeguards the community's clean air, water, food, etc., and has a role to play in controlling notifiable diseases. There is however a Senior community Medical Officer in every District Health Authority, designated to liaise with environmental health officers on any medical problems which may arise.

SECTION II
MULTIPLE RESPONSE QUESTIONS Questions 6.45–6.63

Select any number of correct responses between 1–5.

6.45 The following are among the four major causes of maternal death:
A infection
B pulmonary embolus
C abortion
D haemorrhage
E diabetes mellitus

6.46 The Peel Report on the Maternity Services in 1969, recommended:
A increased domiciliary deliveries
B 100 per cent hospital confinement
C an integrated midwifery service
D male midwives
E abolition of community midwifery services

6.47 Syphilis:
A is treated with metronidazole (Flagyl)
B can be transmitted to the fetus *in utero*
C is caused by a motile spirochaete
D can cause abortion or stillbirth
E produces a large oedematous placenta

6.48 Gonorrhoea in women:
A is characterised by a profuse, painful discharge
B may be detected by culturing cervical and urethral swabs
C is on the increase in the United Kingdom
D causes a primary chancre
E is often masked by candidiasis or trichomoniasis

6.49 The gonococcus is:
A a Gram negative diplococcus
B the causative organism of yaws
C always sensitive to penicillin
D easily cultured from a vaginal swab
E a dangerous cause of ophthalmia neonatorum

6.50 Candida albicans is:
A treated with metronidazole (flagyl)
B a yeast-like fungus
C characterised by flagella
D a common cause of vaginal infections
E frequently seen associated with diabetes

(*answers overleaf*)

6.45 **B C D**
The other main cause of maternal death is severe pre-eclampsia and eclampsia. Infection is now a rare cause of maternal mortality.

6.46 **B C**
Hospital confinement rates are now in the region of 99 per cent, and hospital and domiciliary midwifery services are gradually evolving into a single integrated service.

6.47 **B C D E**
Although the *Treponema pallidum* is a large organism, its motile cork-screw shape allows it to enter the placenta, and infect and damage the fetus during pregnancy. At delivery, the placenta is characteristically large, unhealthy and oedematous.

6.48 **B C E**
Unlike the disease in males, gonorrhoea in women may be largely symptom free. The gonococcus is often difficult to culture, and can be masked by co-existing candidiasis or trichomoniasis.

6.49 **A E**
There are now an increasing number of penicillin resistant gonococci, and other antibiotics may have to be used such as the tetracyclines or kanamycin. The gonococcus is easily destroyed, and can usually only be successfully cultured from cervical, urethral or rectal swabs which are plated and incubated immediately.

6.50 **B D E**
Diabetics with persistent glycosuria, are very prone to candidiasis.

6.51 Notifiable diseases:
- **A** include smallpox, gonococcal ophthalmia neonatorum and tetanus
- **B** have to be notified by a doctor to the District Health Authority
- **C** are dangerous or epidemic diseases
- **D** are notified by a nurse or midwife in charge of the case
- **E** include coryza, influenza and rubella

6.52 When a midwife delivers a stillborn baby, the normal procedure which follows includes:
- **A** immediate removal of the stillbirth to limit the parents' distress
- **B** signing of the death certificate for the parents
- **C** signing of the stillbirth certificate by the doctor or midwife
- **D** instruction to the parents to register the stillbirth and obtain a disposal certificate
- **E** opportunity for the parents to see their stillborn child and work through their grief with midwives and doctors

6.53 The UK Central Council:
- **A** was set up by the 1979 Nurses, Midwives and Health Visitors Act
- **B** inspects nursing homes with a midwifery workload
- **C** carries out general supervision of all practising midwives
- **D** is responsible for framing the rules governing midwifery practice
- **E** approves midwifery training institutions

6.54 The health visitor:
- **A** may staff the School Health Service
- **B** is an expert in preventive health care
- **C** is usually based in a consultant maternity unit
- **D** actively monitors child development in the community
- **E** is a member of the primary health care team

6.55 Social Services Departments:
- **A** administer the Home Help Service
- **B** are administered by the local authority
- **C** provide nursery school education
- **D** provide facilities for the physically and mentally handicapped
- **E** are organised by the National Health Service

(*answers overleaf*)

6.51 **A B C**

Notifiable diseases are notified to the District Health Authority by a *doctor*. The legal responsibility of a midwife (or nurse), is to inform a doctor, and carry out his prescribed treatment.

6.52 **C D E**

Generally, the doctor will sign a stillbirth certificate, but a midwife may do so if she was present at the delivery. It is important to help the parents work through their grief, and see their dead baby if they so wish.

6.53 **A D**

Inspection of nursing homes with a midwifery workload and general supervision of midwives are duties of the local supervising authority. The National Boards undertake the approval of midwifery training institutions.

6.54 **A B D E**

Health visitors are generally based in the community, and many are attached to group practices. However, one health visitor may work as a liaison officer with a consultant maternity unit.

6.55 **A B D**

All local government departments are outside the National Health Service, and nursery school education is provided by the Education Department of the local authority.

6.56 Which of the following statements about the maternity grant are correct?

A a weekly, earnings related payment
B payable for the second twin if it survives for 12 hours of more
C payable on husband's insurance contributions only
D payable when baby is stillborn
E can be claimed up to three months after the birth

6.57 Community Health Councils:

A represent the public in monitoring the quality of the National Health Service
B have one third of their membership appointed by voluntary organisations
C have all members appointed by the Regional Health Authority
D have half their membership appointed by the local authority (local government)
E are appointed in every health district

6.58 Which of the following are approved methods for arranging an adoption?

A third party adoption
B direct adoption
C private adoption
D registered adoption society
E Social Services Department

6.59 When a child is adopted:

A the order has to be granted by a court of law
B the adoption order, once granted, transfers all legal parental rights to the adopters
C a trial period of at least three months must precede the court hearing of the adoption application
D the court appoints a 'guardian *ad litem*' (usually a social worker) for the duration of the 'trial period' to safeguard the child
E the adoptive parents should be at least 21 years old

(*answers overleaf*)

6.56 **B D E**
Is a single lump sum paid to the mother and *not* now linked to National Insurance Contributions. An extra grant is payable to all second or subsequent babies of a multiple pregnancy who survive 12 hours or more

6.57 **A B D E**
The remaining members are appointed by the Regional Health Authority.

6.58 **D E**
Private adoption, either 'direct' or 'third party', is an inadequate method of arranging an adoption, and was discontinued with the implementation of the 1975 Children's Act.

6.59 **A B C D E**

6.60 The unsupported, single parent may:
- **A** suffer social deprivation
- **B** need to place her child in a day nursery
- **C** join a supportive organisation such as 'Gingerbread'
- **D** have inadequate, bad housing
- **E** belong to a low income group

6.61 Which of the following services are provided by the Social Services Department of the local authority?
- **A** fostering
- **B** nursery schools
- **C** child minding
- **D** day nurseries
- **E** children's homes

6.62 Day nurseries:
- **A** give priority to working mothers with social problems
- **B** open five days a week from about 8 a.m.–6 p.m.
- **C** cater for children aged 6 weeks–5 years
- **D** are staffed by RGNs, nursery nurses, etc.
- **E** provide pre-school education through the local education authority

6.63 Prescription Only Medicines:
- **A** are regulated by the Misuse of Drugs Act 1971
- **B** include 'Narcan' (naloxone) and ergometrine
- **C** are legislated for in the Medicines Act 1968
- **D** can only be prescribed by a doctor
- **E** include pethidine and 'Narcan' (naloxone)

(*answers overleaf*)

6.60 **A B C D E**
Single-parent families have multiple problems, often stemming from inadequate finance, and lack of family support.

6.61 **A C D E**
Social Services Departments provide facilities for children whose natural parents cannot or will not give them adequate care and protection.

6.62 **A B C D**
Pre-school education is provided by *nursery schools.*

6.63 **B C**
Prescription Only Medicines are regulated by a section of the Medicines Act 1968, and the limited prescribing rights of community midwives are clearly laid down in this Act. Drugs such as ergometrine, 'Syntometrine', 'Narcan', 'Fortral', and chloral derivatives are listed for use by community midwives in the course of their professional practice.

SECTION III
TRUE OR FALSE? Questions 6.64–6.74

Indicate whether the statements below are true or false.

6.64 **Widespread rubella vaccination is reducing the number of infants born with congenital malformations.**

6.65 **Community midwives are permitted, under the Misuse of Drugs and Medicines Acts, to possess and prescribe, within due limits, pethidine, pentazocine and methadone.**

6.66 **The National Boards approve and regularly inspect all midwifery training schools.**

6.67 **The rules and regulations of the UK Central Council are administered at a local level by the local supervising authority.**

6.68 **The 'trial' period for adoption may begin when the baby is one week old, and must last for a minimum of three months.**

6.69 **The Health Education Council is a national organisation which provides help and advice on health education.**

6.70 **Abortion is no longer the leading cause of maternal death, due to the 1967 Abortion Act.**

6.71 **Abnormal behaviour and lack of maternal affection in the early postnatal period, may be danger signs indicating an increased risk of future child abuse.**

6.72 **The Social Services Department is responsible for providing facilities for the elderly and the handicapped.**

6.73 **All infants should be vaccinated against smallpox before school age.**

6.74 **Caesarean section must never be undertaken when the woman is suffering from acute genital herpes.**

(*answers overleaf*)

6.64 **True**
This is one of the few areas where progress has been made in reducing the incidence of congenital defects.

6.65 **False**
Under the Misuse of Drugs and Medicines Acts, community midwives have limited prescribing rights for pethidine and pentazocine (Fortral), but *not* methadone (Physeptone).

6.66 **True**

6.67 **True**

6.68 **False**
The trial period for the adoption may not begin until the baby is at least *six weeks old*, although many adoptive parents may *foster* the baby when it is 1–2 weeks old until the trial period can commence. The minimum trial period is *three* months, but this can be extended when necessary.

6.69 **True**

6.70 **True**
There has been an enormous reduction in the number of 'back street' abortionists undertaking criminal abortion. However this is not the only factor which has led to greatly decreased numbers of septic abortions and deaths.

6.71 **True**

6.72 **True**

6.73 **False**
The World Health Organisation reports that smallpox is now well controlled throughout the world, and in his country children are no longer routinely vaccinated.

6.74 **False**
Severe genital herpes may be an indication for caesarean section to prevent major infection of the baby during vaginal delivery.

SECTION IV
MATCHING ITEMS Questions 6.75–6.78

Match the items in Group 1 with the most appropriate item in Group 2. (Each item in Group 2 may only be used *once*.)

6.75 Match items in Group 1 with the most appropriate item in Group 2.

Group 1		*Group 2*
(i) rabies	**A**	syphilis
(ii) measles vaccine	**B**	diphtheria, tetanus,
(iii) spirochaete	**C**	whooping cough
(iv) triple vaccine	**C**	12–14 months
	D	notifiable disease
	E	diphtheria, pertussis, measles

6.76 Match the items in Group 1 with the most appropriate item in Group 2.

Group 1		*Group 2*
(i) spermicides	**A**	Dumas cap
(ii) diaphragm 'cap'	**B**	hostile cervical mucus
(iii) progestogen 'mini-pill'	**C**	rhythm method
(iv) 'safe' period	**D**	effective about three hours
	E	must be checked if significant weight loss occurs

6.77 Match the items in Group 1 with the most appropriate item in Group 2.

Group 1		*Group 2*
(i) pemphigus	**A**	live, attenuated virus
(ii) day nurseries	**B**	stillbirths and first week deaths
(iii) poliomyelitis vaccine	**C**	passive immunisation
(iv) perinatal mortality	**D**	*Staphylococcus aureus*
	E	single parent families

6.78 Match the items in Group 1 with the most appropriate item in Group 2.

Group 1		*Group 2*
(i) condom ('sheath')	**A**	prostaglandins
(ii) therapeutic abortion	**B**	guardian *ad litem*
(iii) home confinement	**C**	general practitioner unit
(iv) adoption	**D**	reduced incidence of venereal disease
	E	obstetric 'Flying Squad'

(*answers overleaf*)

6.75
(i) **D**
(ii) **C**
(iii) **A**
(iv) **B**

6.76
(i) **D**
(ii) **E**
(iii) **B**
(iv) **C**

6.77
(i) **D**
(ii) **E**
(iii) **A**
(iv) **B**

6.78
(i) **D**
(ii) **A**
(iii) **E**
(iv) **B**

SECTION V
ASSERTION/REASON Questions 6.79–6.84

Read carefully the five possible answers listed below marked A, B, C, D and E. Select which is appropriate for the assertions and reasons which follow.

A Assertion true; reason is a true statement, and is the correct reason.
B Assertion and reason both true, but reason in *not* the correct reason.
C Assertion is true, but reason is a false statement.
D Assertion is false, but the reason is a true statement.
E Assertion and reason are both false.

6.79 **Health Care Planning Teams have been set up in all Health Districts**
because
they can analyse and assess the needs, and priorities of the health services, and produce a better use of resources.

6.80 **The unsupported mother who works full time cannot usually use a nursery school or play group for her child**
because
she is not eligible for this facility.

6.81 **Gonococcal ophthalmia is the most dangerous eye infection in the neonate**
because
the baby will always contract systemic gonorrhoea

6.82 **all births must be notified to the District Health Authority within 36 hours of birth**
because
the health visitor needs to be informed quickly, so that she may arrange to visit the family by the 10th–12th day.

6.83 **Mothers should be advised against smoking in pregnancy**
because
their babies may suffer from intra-uterine growth retardation.

6.84 **Immunisation against whooping cough is recommended in children with a history of convulsions.**
because
immunisation will be effective in the presence of this condition.

(*answers overleaf*)

6.79 **A**

Health care planning teams are set up in different specialities (e.g. geriatrics, maternity, etc.) in an attempt to plan ahead and utilise resources and finances to the best advantage.

6.80 **C**

The working single parent *is* eligible to use nursery schools or play groups, but they do not care for the child for the whole working day, or during the holidays. Therefore, she needs to use a day nursery or registered child minder.

6.81 **C**

Gonococcal ophthalmia is a dangerous infection because it may, if neglected, lead to blindness. However, the infant does not usually contract systemic gonorrhoea.

6.82 **A**

6.83 **A**

6.84 **D**

Pertussis immunisation *is* effective in children with a history of convulsions, but is *contra-indicated* because of the increased risk of a vaccine encephalitis and possible brain damage.

SECTION VI
COMPLETION ITEMS Questions 6.85–6.95

Supply the missing word(s) in the following statements:

6.85 CASE HISTORY
Sally, an 18-year old single girl, is newly delivered in a maternity hospital, following a concealed pregnancy and no antenatal care. She has no home to go to, but wishes to keep her baby.

Using the above information, supply the appropriate word(s) to the following five statements:

(i) **The midwife in charge of the postnatal ward should arrange for Sally to have an early visit from the____________________________**

(ii) **Following discharge from hospital it is arranged for Sally to stay in a____________________until she finds permanent accommodation.**

(iii) **Sally is a fully-trained secretary, and keen to go back to work, so arrangements are made for the baby to be cared for in a____________________while Sally is at work.**

(iv) **Until she can start work, Sally is very short of money, but as she had been working full time up until a few weeks before she had the baby, she will be entitled to the following financial benefits:**

a ____________________________
b ____________________________
c ____________________________

(v) **Sally states that she is not sure who is the father of her baby. If the mother is certain (and particularly if the father actually admits it), then she can apply to a court of law for a____________________order.**

(*answers overleaf*)

6.85

(i) social worker
(ii) mother and baby home
(iii) day nursery
(iv) a maternity grant
b maternity allowance
c supplementary benefits
(v) paternity/affiliation

6.86 **Chest X-ray in pregnancy may be carried out to exclude ____________. This disease is not common nowadays, but is more likely to occur where there is a large ____________ community.**

6.87 **A child who needs semi-permanent, full-time care, will be accommodated in a children's home or with ____________.**

6.88 **General practitioners, community nurses and midwives, and health visitors form the basis of the ____________.**

6.89 **Adoptions should be arranged through a ____________ or ____________.**

6.90 **The two statutory administrative tiers of the National Health Service are ____________ and ____________.**

6.91 **Toxoids and live vaccines are used to confer ____________ immunity, while antitoxic and convalescent sera may be used to provide ____________ immunity.**

6.92 **____________ is a weekly payment made to all parents to assist with the cost of bringing up their families.**

6.93 **Cot deaths are now more generally referred to as ____________, and occur more commonly in ____________ fed babies.**

6.94 **From September 1983 ____________ were granted equal opportunities to train and practise as midwives, and Health Authorities now have to ensure that there is adequate ____________ for female patients, and that these women can receive care from a ____________ attendant if they so choose.**

6.95 **The committee of inquiry into Human Fertilization and Embryology was chaired by ____________.**

(*answers overleaf*)

6.86 **A** pulmonary tuberculosis
B immigrant

6.87 Foster parents

6.88 Primary health care team

6.89 **A** Registered adoption society
B Social Services Department

6.90 **A** Regional Health Authorities
B District Health Authorities

6.91 **A** Active
B Passive

6.92 Child benefit*

6.93 **A** sudden infant deaths
B artificially (bottle)

6.94 **A** men
B chaperoning
C female

6.95 Dame Mary Warnock
This committee dealt with many aspects of in vitro fertilisation, research using 'spare' embryos and surrogacy.

*The current child benefit for 19______ is £______ per week for each child.

COMMUNITY HEALTH

The following questions are taken from recent examination set by the English National Board.

1. Essay questions

Discuss the factors which may lead to non-accidental injury. List the signs of non-accidental injury. What action would a midwife take if she suspected a baby was being abused? (1983)

Discuss the ways in which a midwife may fulfil her role in advising parents on the protection of their baby from infection, infectious diseases and accidents. (1983)

Outline the arrangements that have to be made for a planned early transfer home. What problems affecting the mother may the community midwife encounter and how should she deal with them? (1983)

Discuss the advice and support that the midwife should give to the parents of a handicapped child. (1983)

Women should have the right to choose where they will be confined and the total management they receive.
Discuss this statement with particular emphasis on labour and delivery. (1983)

In accordance with the Midwives Rules the midwife is required to keep detailed records of all cases she attends. What records are kept during pregnancy and labour? Discuss the need for and the significance of these records. (1983)

An unbooked, multigravid woman, who is in established labour at term, calls a midwife to her home. The breech is found to be presenting. How is this confirmed?
Discuss the midwife's management including her delivery of the baby. (1984)

A newly delivered mother is considering offering her baby for adoption. Describe the special skills required of the midwife. What knowledge of other services will help the midwife to meet the total needs of this woman? (1984)

List the recent causes of maternal mortality.
What factors have influenced the decline in this mortality rate during the last 40 years? (1984)

Discuss the care and support that should be offered by the midwife to a pregnant 14-year-old and her family (1984)

Describe the services available from birth to 1 year to promote positive health and detect any abnormalities. (1984)

Define perinatal mortality. List the main causes of perinatal death. In what ways can parents, health professionals and voluntary organisations work together to reduce the perinatal death rate? (1985)

2. Write briefly on each of the following subjects?
Value of Child Health Clinics (1983)
Main causes of maternal mortality (1983)
Notification and registration of birth (1983)
Role of the Supervisor of Midwives (1983)
Day care facilities for the under 5-year-olds (1983)
Rubella vaccination (1983)
Alternatives to a mother's care (1983)
Follow up of a normal baby from the 10th day of life (1983)
Perinatal mortality (1983)
Fetal Alcohol Syndrome (1983)
Notification of intention to practise (1984)
Statutory duties of a midwife during the postnatal period (1984)
Sudden infant death (cot death) (1984)
Sibling rivalry (1984)
Liaison between midwives and health visitors (1984)
Unemployed fathers (1984)
Drug abuse during pregnancy (1984)
Neonatal mortality (1984)
Immunisation programme (1985)
Genetic counselling (1985)
Surrogate mothers (1985)
The 'Warnock Report' (1985)
Rules and regulations relating to Controlled Drugs (1985)
Acquired Immune Deficiency Syndrome (AIDS) (1985)
The law in relation to termination of pregnancy (1985)

References and further reading

Adams M, Prince J 1978 Minds, mothers and midwives. Churchill Livingstone, Edinburgh

Baker A A 1967 Psychiatric disorders in obstetrics. Blackwell Scientific Publications, Oxford

Barnes C G 1976 Medical disorders in obstetric practice. Blackwell Scientific Publications, Oxford

Balaskas J, Balaskas A 1983 New life. Sidgwick and Jackson, London

Beischer N A, Mackay E V 1976 Obstetrics and the newborn. Holt-Saunders Ltd, Eastbourne

Bertzin N 1981 The gentle birth book. John Murray, London

Brown R J K, Valman H B 1979 Practical neonatal paediatrics, 2nd edn. Blackwell Scientific Publications, Oxford

Burnett/Anderson 1979 Anatomy and physiology of obstetrics. Faber and Faber, London

Davies P A, Robinson L J, Scopes J W, Tizard J P M, Wigglesworth J W 1978 Medical care of newborn babies. Heinemann (William) Medical Books Ltd, London

Donald I 1979 Practical obstetric problems, 5th edn, Lloyd-Luke (Medical Books) Ltd, London

Garrey M M, Govan A D T, Hodge C, Callander R 1980 Obstetrics illustrated, 3rd edn. Churchill livingstone, Edinburgh

Grundy F 1974 Community health and social services. Lewis HK and Co Ltd, London

Guide to the social services 1984 Family Welfare Association, London

James D E 1972 A student's guide to efficient study. Pergamon Press, Oxford

Keay A J, Morgan D M 1982 Craig's care of the newly born infant, 7th edn. Churchill Livingstone, Edinburgh

Kitzinger S 1972 The experience of childbirth. Penguin Books, Harmondsworth

Klaus M H, Kennell J H 1982 Parent-infant bonding. C V Mosby Co, Toronto

Korones S 1981 High risk newborn infants, 3rd edn. C V Mosby Co, Toronto

Leboyer F 1975 Birth without violence. Wildwood House Ltd, London

Llewellyn-Jones D 1982 Fundamentals of obstetrics and gynaecology, vol 1 Obstetrics. Faber and Faber, London

Loudon N 1985 Handbook of family planning. Churchill Livingstone, Edinburgh

MacKeith R, Wood C 1982 Infant feeding and difficulties. Churchill Livingstone, Edinburgh

McClure Brown J C, Dixon G 1978 Browne's antenatal care, 11th edn. Churchill Livingstone, Edinburgh

Meredith Davies J B 1983, 5th edn. Community health, preventive medicine and social services. Ballière Tindall, London

Moin D 1982 Pain relief in labour, 4th edn. Churchill Livingstone, Edinburgh

Myles M F 1985 A textbook for midwives, 10th edn. Churchill Livingstone, Edinburgh

Rowntree D 1970 Learn how to study. MacDonald and Jane's Publishers Ltd, London

Siggers D 1978 Prenatal diagnosis of genetic disease. Blackwell Scientific Publications, Oxford

Stanley P, Stanley A 1978 Breast is best. Pan Books, London

Sweet B 1982 Mayes midwifery. Ballière Tindall, London

Verralls S 1979 Anatomy applied to obstetrics. Pitman Medical Publishing Co Ltd, Tunbridge Wells

Vulliamy D 1982 The newborn child, 4th edn. Churchill Livingstone, Edinburgh

Williams M, Booth D 1985 Antenatal education and guidelines for teachers, 3rd edn. Churchill Livingstone, Edinburgh